RUNNER'S WORLD®
TRAINING
JOURNAL

Name: _____

Address: _____

Journal for the Year _____ to _____

© 2012 by Rodale Inc.

Rodale books may be purchased for business or promotional use or for special sales. For information, please write to:
Special Markets Department, Rodale, Inc., 733 Third Avenue, New York, NY 10017

Runner's World* is a registered trademark of Rodale Inc.

Printed in China
Rodale Inc. makes every effort to use acid-free ♾, recycled paper ♻.

Photo Credits for interior photographs are listed on page 174.
Book design by Christopher Rhoads

ISBN 978–1–60961–854–4 paperback

Distributed to the trade by Macmillan
6 8 10 9 7 5 paperback

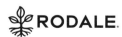

We inspire and enable people to improve their lives and the world around them.
www.rodalebooks.com

CONTENTS

INTRODUCTION

When my running buddies discover my vast trove of training journals (40 years' worth) on a dusty bookshelf, they can rarely suppress their laughter. You see, I have obsessive tendencies. There, I said it. Admitting it is the first step, right?

One training journal page explains how I once ran sixty 200-meter repeats on an indoor track. It was February in New England, as I recall—a good time to be indoors. The workout wasn't actually as hard as it might sound. After the first half-dozen repeats, I got into a groove, a trance of sorts. The next 54 passed like a dream.

When I had injuries, my journal entries switched gears, turning to desperate attempts at rehabilitation. A throbbing Achilles tendon just about drove me to madness. I had a big race coming up—big, as in a 54-mile-long ultramarathon—and my swollen Achilles wouldn't even permit a short hobble. I decided masochism must be the answer, icing the afflicted area once an hour, followed each time by squeezing the tendon as hard as I could. This was roughly the equivalent of hitting myself on the thumb with a hammer. Amazingly, it worked; I was able to finish the ultramarathon.

A runner's training journal, like the one in your hands, has many potential uses. You can scribble in the margins, as I sometimes did, to explicate the infinite—and sometimes infinitely silly—details of your life. Or you can distill your thoughts and actions first, giving more focus and perhaps more meaning. Since you are a runner, you will no doubt use this journal primarily to record various aspects of your running. Here are four great areas to consider for your daily notes. Any one of them alone can help make you a better, healthier runner. Combine a few, and you'll have enough power to take your running to a whole new level.

MOTIVATION. A training journal should motivate you to run more, or at least more regularly. Indeed, published medical studies have shown that exercise logs are one of the few proven ways to make yourself stick to your goals. Look at those yawning, empty pages. They just beg to be filled in. Don't let them go hungry.

NUTRITION. Training journals are useful for planning and keeping track of how you fuel your body for runs and what foods work best in helping you achieve your goals. Most runners want to combine a good diet with a consistent exercise program. After all, it doesn't make much sense to run 20 miles a week and then undo all the health benefits of a regular aerobic-training program by eating burgers and fries at every meal.

TRAINING AND RACING. Now we've reached the heart of the training journal, the reason you're using one in the first place—to record and analyze your daily, weekly, and yearly training and racing achievements. As you look back over your journal to analyze what worked and what didn't, keep these key principles in mind:

1. Your training should increase gradually for 6 to 16 weeks before major races, particularly before marathons.
2. Even these "buildups" should include easy days and, often, easy weeks.
3. You should taper for 1 to 3 weeks before a big race.
4. You need at least two recovery periods during the year (most people take them during the worst summer heat and during the end-of-year holiday season), during which you dramatically decrease your training for 2 to 4 weeks.
5. You should plan new and different training/racing goals every year to stay fresh and motivated.

INJURY PREVENTION. Runners get injured. That's the bad news. The good news? Most of these injuries are minor muscle and tendon strains that heal quickly if you let them. I repeat: "If you let them." So the first rule of injury prevention is always to take 2 to 4 days off from running at the onset of any running-related pains. You can walk, swim (or pool jog), or perhaps ride your bike. But don't run. The old aphorism "A stitch in time saves nine" applies perfectly to running. Beyond appropriate days off, use ice to limit inflammation, stretch gently after workouts (but not before—a thorough warmup is a much better idea), and do strengthening exercises to build balanced leg muscles. Keep track of your injuries and your methods for rehabbing them in your journal so you can refer to it should the same injury crop up again.

Amby Burfoot
Winner of the 1968 Boston Marathon,
Editor-at-large, *Runner's World*

HOW TO USE THIS JOURNAL

A running journal is more than an account of how many miles you've covered—it's an excellent training tool. Recording details of your runs can keep you on track and excited about your goals, as well as help head off injury. The goal here is to record the information you'll need to help you improve your running and to see what worked and what didn't. Training logs help you stay fit, focused, and motivated.

Even if you write down nothing else, record your mileage or time and how you felt after each run. In addition, try to add a few extra words to the weekly "Notes" section. Here are some suggestions for topics you may want to write about in your journal.

Your Run

MILEAGE OR TIME: Watching the miles, or time, add up can be the most satisfying part of record keeping.

ROUTES AND TERRAIN: Record hills, trail conditions, and surface type (macadam, dirt road, etc.).

INTERVAL OR RACE TIMES: Take a look at your watch at the beginning and end of your run, and note your splits during your run. This will help you monitor your progress.

TEMPERATURE: Temps over 75°F or below 0°F can affect your performance. (Visit runnersworld.com/whattowear for tips on what to wear.)

TIME OF DAY: Body rhythms and the time of day or night may dictate your energy level—we naturally have more energy during certain times of the day. It's different for everyone, and journaling will help you see your own patterns.

PARTNERS: If you join a running club or find a fellow runner, here's the place for their contact info so you can make plans for future runs.

GOALS: Setting targets will give you a sense of purpose. Plan a series of daily, weekly, and monthly objectives.

FUN: Yep, fun! Running can be about fitness and health or setting a PR, but it should also—at least some of the time—be about having fun. Writing down something that made you smile during a run can help you reconnect with the feeling when you get mired in less-than-inspiring concerns. Some of your best ideas may hit you during a run. Did you sing out loud? Skip instead of sprint? Run to your favorite coffeehouse? Enjoy a long run with a good friend or partner? Write it down. Looking back at the fun reinforces how much running enriches your life.

Your Body

ACHES OR PAINS: Record any soreness (no matter where) you felt before, during, or after your run. Notice the patterns. Hard running surfaces or a rapid increase in speedwork miles can sometimes increase your risk of injury. If you are feeling achy, take a rest day, or switch some of your runs to soft surfaces to lessen the impact.

MOOD: Note how you feel before, during, and after a run. To prevent boredom, you can try a new route, join a running group, or take a couple days off.

FOOD: Write down what you ate before and during a run. If you occasionally suffer from GI upset, this will help you identify and avoid troublesome foods or figure out when you should or should not eat relative to going for a run.

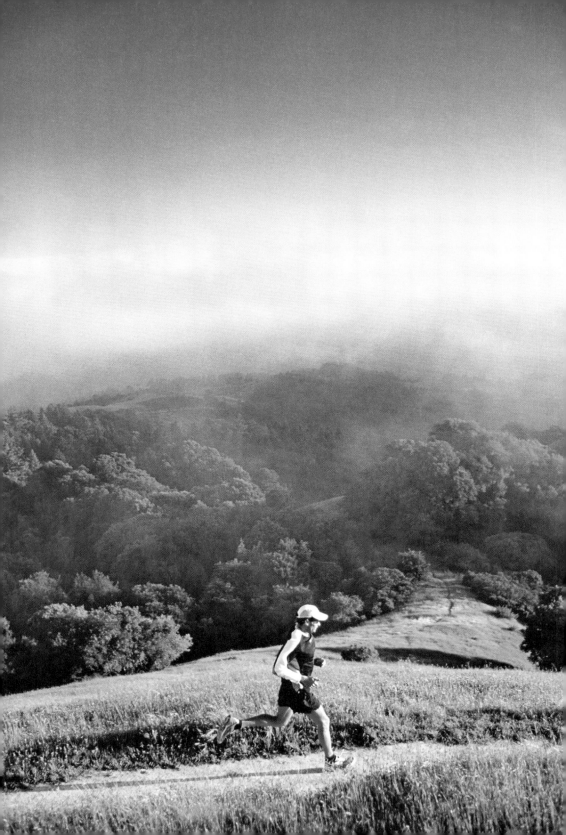

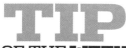

OF THE **WEEK**

Register for a race. Once you put a date on a calendar and pay the entry fee, you are committing yourself to a goal. Having that goal on the horizon will help you motivate on days when you're having a tough time getting moving.

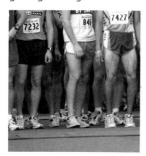

"If you want to become the best runner you can be, start now. Don't spend the rest of your life wondering if you can do it."

—PRISCILLA WELCH,
British Olympic marathoner, winner 1987 New York City Marathon (at age 42)

MONDAY
ROUTE:

DISTANCE: TIME:

NOTES:

CROSS TRAINING:

TUESDAY
ROUTE:

DISTANCE: TIME:

NOTES:

CROSS TRAINING:

WEDNESDAY
ROUTE:

DISTANCE: TIME:

NOTES:

CROSS TRAINING:

THURSDAY
ROUTE:

DISTANCE: TIME:

NOTES:

CROSS TRAINING:

FRIDAY
ROUTE:

DISTANCE: TIME:

NOTES:

CROSS TRAINING:

SATURDAY

ROUTE:

DISTANCE: **TIME:**

NOTES:

CROSS TRAINING:

SUNDAY

ROUTE:

DISTANCE: **TIME:**

NOTES:

CROSS TRAINING:

NOTES

WEEKLY TOTAL

TOTAL MILEAGE TO DATE

NUTRITION

CAFFEINE BOOST!

Many runners rely on a pre-run cup of coffee for an energy boost and to get the GI tract moving, and that's okay. Research has shown that caffeine lowers fatigue and perceived exertion, increases speed, and boosts mood, endurance, and energy, and can boost performance. While it has long been thought that caffeine leads to dehydration, recent research suggests that might not be the case.

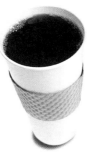

DID YOU KNOW?

The ideal number of steps per minute is 180, no matter your pace.

TIP OF THE **WEEK**

Side stitches are sharp pains usually felt just below the rib cage. For a quick fix, notice which foot is striking the ground when you inhale and exhale, then switch the pattern. (So if you were breathing and leading with your right foot, inhale when your left foot steps.) If that doesn't help, stop running and reach both arms above your head. Bend at the waist, leaning toward the side opposite the stitch.

"For me, running has also been a vehicle of introduction to people, places, cultures, and animals. I have run on all seven continents, but it's not the details of the races I recall, it's the people I meet."

—BART YASSO,
Runner's World chief running officer; winner, 1998 Smoky Mountain Marathon; creator of marathon training tool, Yasso 800s

MONDAY
ROUTE:

DISTANCE:　　　　　　　　　　TIME:

NOTES:

CROSS TRAINING:

TUESDAY
ROUTE:

DISTANCE:　　　　　　　　　　TIME:

NOTES:

CROSS TRAINING:

WEDNESDAY
ROUTE:

DISTANCE:　　　　　　　　　　TIME:

NOTES:

CROSS TRAINING:

THURSDAY
ROUTE:

DISTANCE:　　　　　　　　　　TIME:

NOTES:

CROSS TRAINING:

FRIDAY
ROUTE:

DISTANCE:　　　　　　　　　　TIME:

NOTES:

CROSS TRAINING:

SATURDAY

ROUTE:

DISTANCE: TIME:

NOTES:

CROSS TRAINING:

SUNDAY

ROUTE:

DISTANCE: TIME:

NOTES:

CROSS TRAINING:

NOTES

WEEKLY TOTAL

TOTAL MILEAGE TO DATE

TRAINING

MENTAL SECRETS

At regular intervals as you run, ask yourself how your body feels, whether your rhythm is smooth, and whether your legs can handle the speed. When your mind drifts to other thoughts, simply remind yourself to pay attention. You don't have to micromanage your body 100 percent of the time; be able to shift in and out when you need to focus on the road.

DID YOU KNOW?

Roberta (aka Bobbi) Gibb is recognized as the first woman who ran, albeit unregistered, an entire marathon, in 1966. Kathrine Switzer beat the system in 1967 by registering as K.V. Switzer and ran the Boston Marathon from start to finish.

TIP
OF THE **WEEK**

Don't skip the cooldown, even on slow days. Even if you went out for a casual run, blood can still pool in your legs and cause cramps if you don't cool down. Alternate 30 to 60 seconds of slow running with the same amount of walking for a total of 5 minutes; then walk the final 5 minutes.

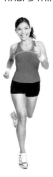

"Sometimes pushing harder is not the answer. It takes self-control, confidence, and intuition to know when to train and when to rest, but when in question, err on the side of being overrested."

—RYAN HALL, Olympic marathoner

MONDAY
ROUTE:

DISTANCE: TIME:

NOTES:

CROSS TRAINING:

TUESDAY
ROUTE:

DISTANCE: TIME:

NOTES:

CROSS TRAINING:

WEDNESDAY
ROUTE:

DISTANCE: TIME:

NOTES:

CROSS TRAINING:

THURSDAY
ROUTE:

DISTANCE: TIME:

NOTES:

CROSS TRAINING:

FRIDAY
ROUTE:

DISTANCE: TIME:

NOTES:

CROSS TRAINING:

SATURDAY

ROUTE:

DISTANCE: TIME:

NOTES:

CROSS TRAINING:

SUNDAY

ROUTE:

DISTANCE: TIME:

NOTES:

CROSS TRAINING:

NOTES

WEEKLY TOTAL

TOTAL MILEAGE TO DATE

NUTRITION

GO ORGANIC

A handful of fruits and vegetables—including spinach, apples, peaches, and strawberries—tend to have particularly high levels of pesticide residues, so organic may be your safest bet. If you can't buy them organic, take extra care when washing these foods.

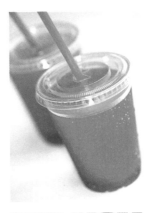

DID YOU KNOW?

In a study conducted by New Zealand researchers, runners who slurped an icy slushy before a sweltering run lasted an average of 10 minutes longer than participants who gulped a cold drink.

TIP
OF THE **WEEK**

Runners who rinsed their mouths with a carb solution right before and every 15 minutes during hour-long treadmill sessions ran faster and about 200 meters farther than those who rinsed with a placebo. For shorter runs, when you want the benefits of a sports drink minus the extra calories, swishing just might be enough.

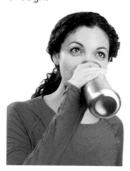

"I want to run with the lead pack . . . you have to be up there in order to win."

—DANIEL NJENGA MUTURI,
Kenyan marathoner; winner 2007 Tokyo and 2009 Hokkaido Marathons

MONDAY
ROUTE:

DISTANCE: TIME:

NOTES:

CROSS TRAINING:

TUESDAY
ROUTE:

DISTANCE: TIME:

NOTES:

CROSS TRAINING:

WEDNESDAY
ROUTE:

DISTANCE: TIME:

NOTES:

CROSS TRAINING:

THURSDAY
ROUTE:

DISTANCE: TIME:

NOTES:

CROSS TRAINING:

FRIDAY
ROUTE:

DISTANCE: TIME:

NOTES:

CROSS TRAINING:

SATURDAY

ROUTE:

DISTANCE: TIME:

NOTES:

CROSS TRAINING:

SUNDAY

ROUTE:

DISTANCE: TIME:

NOTES:

CROSS TRAINING:

NOTES

WEEKLY TOTAL

TOTAL MILEAGE TO DATE

TRAINING

FIX YOUR FORM

Good form can help you run more efficiently, and feel more relaxed on the road. Look straight ahead, not down at your feet. Drop your shoulders, and don't let them creep up to your ears. If you tense up, shake out your hands and arms. Run tall, and don't let yourself crouch over. Keep your hands in an unclenched fist, with your fingers lightly touching your palms, as if you're carrying a piece of paper.

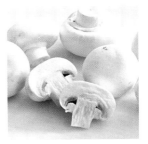

DID YOU KNOW?

Mushrooms are a great source of vitamin D. About 3 ounces contain 400 international units (IU) of vitamin D.

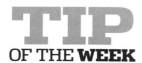

OF THE **WEEK**

Running on a treadmill is a great alternative when the weather conditions make running outside impossible. And there are benefits too: you can also monitor the thermostat, tackle made-to-order hills, and enjoy cushioning that protects your joints. Most important, you force yourself to stick to a pace. Just make sure you vary your workouts. Do a steady run one day, and intervals the next. If you get locked into a routine, your body will adapt and you won't keep building your fitness.

"During my first marathon I was hurting. I was mad. I was angry. I said: 'Never again!'"

—GRETE WAITZ, Norwegian marathoner, 9-time winner of the New York City Marathon, 2-time winner of the London Marathon, Olympic silver medalist (Los Angeles 1984).

MONDAY
ROUTE:

DISTANCE: TIME:

NOTES:

CROSS TRAINING:

TUESDAY
ROUTE:

DISTANCE: TIME:

NOTES:

CROSS TRAINING:

WEDNESDAY
ROUTE:

DISTANCE: TIME:

NOTES:

CROSS TRAINING:

THURSDAY
ROUTE:

DISTANCE: TIME:

NOTES:

CROSS TRAINING:

FRIDAY
ROUTE:

DISTANCE: TIME:

NOTES:

CROSS TRAINING:

SATURDAY

ROUTE:

DISTANCE: **TIME:**

NOTES:

CROSS TRAINING:

SUNDAY

ROUTE:

DISTANCE: **TIME:**

NOTES:

CROSS TRAINING:

NOTES

WEEKLY TOTAL

TOTAL MILEAGE TO DATE

NUTRITION

SWEET TREATS

If you like a sweet treat, it's okay to indulge from time to time. Just be sure to keep it under 250 calories. Here are some options that fit the bill: 10 Hershey's Kisses, 12 Starbursts, 25 Peanut M&Ms, or 40 candy corn pieces.

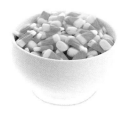

DID YOU KNOW?

The Marathon des Sables runs across 151 miles of the Sahara Desert in Morocco and lasts 6 days. Temperatures can exceed 120°F. Simply finishing is an epic achievement.

TIP
OF THE **WEEK**

A little speedwork can help you to run faster and smoother. Try a fartlek (Swedish for "speed play") workout that alternates fast, medium, and slow running over a variety of distances. After a steady warmup, simply pick a landmark—a tree, street light, or road sign—and run to it, hard. Once you've reached it, jog until you've recovered. Then pick another landmark, run hard to that, recover, and so on. Go for at least three landmarks.

"Ask yourself: 'Can I give more?' The answer is usually yes."

—PAUL TERGAT, Kenyan marathon; former world record holder (2:04.55) 2003–2007; winner of the New York City Marathon in 2005

MONDAY
ROUTE:

DISTANCE: TIME:

NOTES:

CROSS TRAINING:

TUESDAY
ROUTE:

DISTANCE: TIME:

NOTES:

CROSS TRAINING:

WEDNESDAY
ROUTE:

DISTANCE: TIME:

NOTES:

CROSS TRAINING:

THURSDAY
ROUTE:

DISTANCE: TIME:

NOTES:

CROSS TRAINING:

FRIDAY
ROUTE:

DISTANCE: TIME:

NOTES:

CROSS TRAINING:

SATURDAY

ROUTE:

DISTANCE: TIME:

NOTES:

CROSS TRAINING:

SUNDAY

ROUTE:

DISTANCE: TIME:

NOTES:

CROSS TRAINING:

NOTES

WEEKLY TOTAL

TOTAL MILEAGE TO DATE

TRAINING

EASE INTO IT

Most overuse injuries, from shin splints to IT band syndrome, come from adding too much speed or distance before your body is ready. To stay healthy, build your weekly training mileage by no more than 10 percent per week.

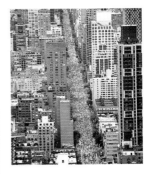

DID YOU KNOW?

The largest marathon (by number of finishers) is the New York City Marathon. It's usually held on the first Sunday in November.

TIP
OF THE **WEEK**

Think of your brain as a carb hog. When your brain is starved, neurons in the occipital cortex misrepresent incoming images. It could make up things that don't even exist: Falling snowflakes become little green men. Some people incorporate them into their consciousness, like a dream state, which is not a good state to be in when you're running a race. Sports drinks that provide as little as 50 grams of carbohydrates can bring your brain back to normal in 10 to 15 minutes.

"A lot of people run a race to see who's the fastest. I run to see who has the most guts."

—STEVE PREFONTAINE,
middle and distance runner;
Olympian in 5,000 m
(Munich 1972)

MONDAY
ROUTE:

DISTANCE: TIME:

NOTES:

CROSS TRAINING:

TUESDAY
ROUTE:

DISTANCE: TIME:

NOTES:

CROSS TRAINING:

WEDNESDAY
ROUTE:

DISTANCE: TIME:

NOTES:

CROSS TRAINING:

THURSDAY
ROUTE:

DISTANCE: TIME:

NOTES:

CROSS TRAINING:

FRIDAY
ROUTE:

DISTANCE: TIME:

NOTES:

CROSS TRAINING:

SATURDAY

ROUTE:

DISTANCE: TIME:

NOTES:

CROSS TRAINING:

SUNDAY

ROUTE:

DISTANCE: TIME:

NOTES:

CROSS TRAINING:

NOTES

WEEKLY TOTAL

TOTAL MILEAGE TO DATE

NUTRITION

THE BEST CHOCOLATE

Need a chocolate fix? Go for dark varieties. Dark chocolate is differentiated by the percentage of cocoa it contains. The higher the percentage, the more cocoa and the less sugar it has. Choose a percentage of 70 or more for the most anti-oxidants. Quality chocolate is made with cocoa butter and milk fat. If vegetable oil, hydrogenated oil, or trans fats are included, skip it.

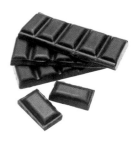

DID YOU KNOW?

In 2010, the men's field for the October 10th Bank of America Chicago Marathon was the most competitive in the event's history—four entrants had run faster than 2:06.

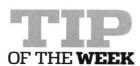

OF THE **WEEK**

When faced with a race-day setback—whether it's one you wake up with (upset stomach) or one that comes midstride (muscle cramps)—there's a decision to make. Since you've trained long and hard for the event, be it a 10-K or a marathon, it's likely to be a tough one. If you drop out, you might be racked by regrets. But bowing out can prevent a small issue from becoming a serious one. If you feel something that's sharp, piercing, or stabbing, slow down to see if it subsides. If it persists or it intensifies, walk to an aid station or wait for medical help to come to you. Pain, pressure, or tightness in your chest are symptoms that demand immediate attention.

"The primary reason to have a coach is to have somebody who can look at you and say, 'Man, you're looking good today.'"

—JACK DANIELS, coach and author of *Daniels' Running Formula*

MONDAY
ROUTE:

DISTANCE: TIME:

NOTES:

CROSS TRAINING:

TUESDAY
ROUTE:

DISTANCE: TIME:

NOTES:

CROSS TRAINING:

WEDNESDAY
ROUTE:

DISTANCE: TIME:

NOTES:

CROSS TRAINING:

THURSDAY
ROUTE:

DISTANCE: TIME:

NOTES:

CROSS TRAINING:

FRIDAY
ROUTE:

DISTANCE: TIME:

NOTES:

CROSS TRAINING:

SATURDAY

ROUTE:

DISTANCE: TIME:

NOTES:

CROSS TRAINING:

SUNDAY

ROUTE:

DISTANCE: TIME:

NOTES:

CROSS TRAINING:

NOTES

WEEKLY TOTAL

TOTAL MILEAGE TO DATE

TRAINING

FEET TREATS

Some runners are particularly prone to dry skin, which invariably leads to painful, cracking feet. Use a moisturizer such as a foot cream every day. Rub it into your skin until your feet feel soft and smooth. The best time to moisturize your feet is immediately after a bath or shower. Applying moisturizer at that time will help retain some of the water from your shower. For those especially prone to blisters, use a skin moisturizer or lubricant on the skin, and also outside your sock, to cut down on the friction that causes blisters. Various brands of petroleum jelly work well, as do non-petroleum-based sport products such as Bodyglide.

DID YOU KNOW?

Bill Bowerman and Nike, Inc., are co-holders of the first patent on the waffle sole for running shoes. Bill got his inspiration from—you guessed it—his wife's waffle iron.

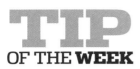

OF THE **WEEK**

Glancing at a small object that reminds you of why you're running can motivate you and ease race-day jitters. Choose something small that has sentimental value and can be carried or worn without hindering your stride.

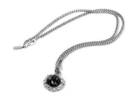

"I thrive on being a part of something bigger than myself . . . I love contributing to a team. I enjoy sharing the process and the outcome. It is much more fun to celebrate this wonderful sport with others!"

—SHALANE FLANAGAN,
distance and marathon runner, Olympic 10,000 m bronze medalist (Beijing 2008)

MONDAY
ROUTE:

DISTANCE: TIME:

NOTES:

CROSS TRAINING:

TUESDAY
ROUTE:

DISTANCE: TIME:

NOTES:

CROSS TRAINING:

WEDNESDAY
ROUTE:

DISTANCE: TIME:

NOTES:

CROSS TRAINING:

THURSDAY
ROUTE:

DISTANCE: TIME:

NOTES:

CROSS TRAINING:

FRIDAY
ROUTE:

DISTANCE: TIME:

NOTES:

CROSS TRAINING:

SATURDAY

ROUTE:

DISTANCE: TIME:

NOTES:

CROSS TRAINING:

SUNDAY

ROUTE:

DISTANCE: TIME:

NOTES:

CROSS TRAINING:

NOTES

WEEKLY TOTAL

TOTAL MILEAGE TO DATE

NUTRITION

GOING VEG

If you're going to forsake all animal products, think about protein-rich plant foods at every meal. It's possible to get 75 to 105 grams of protein a day by eating a variety of soy products, beans, legumes, nuts, and whole grains, as long as you pay close attention to what you're eating. Add a little peanut butter to your bagel, toss some lentils into your pasta sauce, or add chickpeas to a salad. Also, protein in bread, cereal, and grains can add up. Hint: Make changes slowly. A hummus, cheese, and veggie sandwich one day, a turkey sandwich the next. Cottage cheese or yogurt for breakfast on Tuesday, low-fat bacon on Wednesday. A gradual switch will help keep your energy levels high.

DID YOU KNOW?

On race day, crowding at water stops can suck up valuable time. Run to the last or second-to-last table, make eye contact with the volunteers, and grab the cup.

TIP
OF THE **WEEK**

Skin-against-skin and skin-against-clothing rubbing can cause a red, raw rash that can bleed and sting. Moisture and salt on the body make it worse. The underarms, inner thighs, along the bra line (for women), and the nipples (for men) are vulnerable spots. Wear moisture-wicking, seamless, tagless gear. Fit is important—a baggy shirt has excess material that can cause irritation; a too-snug sports bra can dig into skin. Apply Vaseline, sports lube, Band-Aids, or Nip-Guards before you run. And moisturize—drier skin tends to chafe more.

"Distance is one of the only things in life you truly earn."

—MARC PARENT,
the newbie chronicles columnist
for *Runner's World*

MONDAY
ROUTE:

DISTANCE: TIME:

NOTES:

CROSS TRAINING:

TUESDAY
ROUTE:

DISTANCE: TIME:

NOTES:

CROSS TRAINING:

WEDNESDAY
ROUTE:

DISTANCE: TIME:

NOTES:

CROSS TRAINING:

THURSDAY
ROUTE:

DISTANCE: TIME:

NOTES:

CROSS TRAINING:

FRIDAY
ROUTE:

DISTANCE: TIME:

NOTES:

CROSS TRAINING:

SATURDAY

ROUTE:

DISTANCE: TIME:

NOTES:

CROSS TRAINING:

SUNDAY

ROUTE:

DISTANCE: TIME:

NOTES:

CROSS TRAINING:

NOTES

WEEKLY TOTAL

TOTAL MILEAGE TO DATE

TRAINING

TALK TEST

You can use the talk test to make sure you're running at the right level of intensity. On an easy run, for instance, you want to be running comfortably enough that you can hold a conversation. That is at a steady aerobic level, which roughly corresponds to about 65 to 75 percent of your maximum heart rate. If you're huffing and puffing on an easy run, you're going too fast. If you're running at marathon pace, you should be able to speak in full sentences. If you're on a tempo run, a few words at a time may be all you're able to manage. But if you're doing speedwork, you'll just be able to say one word at a time.

DID YOU KNOW?

Approximately 3 percent of Americans follow a strict plant-based diet. And about 25 percent of Americans eat a diet high in fruits and vegetables and low in animal-based foods, according to the American Dietetic Association, a trend called flexitarianism.

TIP
OF THE **WEEK**

The type of canine running buddy you should choose depends on what type of runner you are. If you run 5 to 10 miles at 8-minute pace or faster, you'll want a dog who's athletic, energetic, and built for speed. Here are some pointers.

1. Dogs best suited for running—at any pace—are those who are above knee height. You're likely to trip over dogs who are shorter, even if they heel well.

2. Breeds such as German shorthaired (and wire-haired) pointers, vizslas, and Weimaraners make superb runners. They tend to be able to go long distances—over 10 miles. They find that trot and just keep going straight ahead, oblivious to distractions.

3. Herding dogs (border collies, Australian shepherds, kelpies) and standard poodles between 30 to 60 pounds generally are athletic enough to run well, as are cattle dogs.

NOTE: Labs make good runners, but those with brown or black coats can overheat quickly in warm weather.

MONDAY
ROUTE:

DISTANCE: TIME:

NOTES:

CROSS TRAINING:

TUESDAY
ROUTE:

DISTANCE: TIME:

NOTES:

CROSS TRAINING:

WEDNESDAY
ROUTE:

DISTANCE: TIME:

NOTES:

CROSS TRAINING:

THURSDAY
ROUTE:

DISTANCE: TIME:

NOTES:

CROSS TRAINING:

FRIDAY
ROUTE:

DISTANCE: TIME:

NOTES:

CROSS TRAINING:

SATURDAY
ROUTE:

DISTANCE: TIME:

NOTES:

CROSS TRAINING:

SUNDAY
ROUTE:

DISTANCE: TIME:

NOTES:

CROSS TRAINING:

NOTES

WEEKLY TOTAL

TOTAL MILEAGE TO DATE

NUTRITION

PROTEIN POWER

To repair muscle fibers damaged during strength training, eat lean protein sources. Fat-free dairy, soy products, fish, lean beef, poultry, and eggs all supply needed amino acids. Aim for approximately 80 grams of protein per day.

"I've always taken the philosophy that you have to dream a little in this sport . . . if you stay in your comfort zone, you're not going to do anything special."

—DEENA KASTOR,
marathoner, Olympic bronze medalist (Athens 2004)

DID YOU KNOW?

Fifty percent of respondents to a *Runner's World* poll said that when lining up for a race, they thought they could've trained harder. Some probably *could* have prepared better, but negative thinking is counterproductive. Remind yourself of the training you have done and review your race plan.

TIP
OF THE **WEEK**

Sore from a long run? Try a DIY massage. Start by squeezing each toe on one foot, then squeeze your Achilles tendon a few times. As you work up your leg, intensify the pressure on your calves and quads. Squeeze your muscles with one or both hands, or press into them with your fist or elbow. Repeat on your other leg.

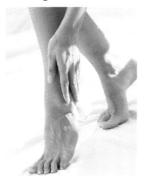

"Do the work. Do the analysis. But feel your run. Feel your race. Feel the joy that is running."

—KARA GOUCHER,
Olympic marathoner, winner of the 10,000 m and bronze medalist at the 2007 World Championships

MONDAY
ROUTE:

DISTANCE: TIME:

NOTES:

CROSS TRAINING:

TUESDAY
ROUTE:

DISTANCE: TIME:

NOTES:

CROSS TRAINING:

WEDNESDAY
ROUTE:

DISTANCE: TIME:

NOTES:

CROSS TRAINING:

THURSDAY
ROUTE:

DISTANCE: TIME:

NOTES:

CROSS TRAINING:

FRIDAY
ROUTE:

DISTANCE: TIME:

NOTES:

CROSS TRAINING:

SATURDAY

ROUTE:

DISTANCE: TIME:

NOTES:

CROSS TRAINING:

SUNDAY

ROUTE:

DISTANCE: TIME:

NOTES:

CROSS TRAINING:

NOTES

WEEKLY TOTAL

TOTAL MILEAGE TO DATE

TRAINING

WINTER TRAINING

When winter blows in, there's no reason to cancel your run. Just dress right, cover your extremities, stay dry, and keep moving. Studies have shown that if you're exercising at 60 percent of VO2 max—a level of intensity you'd maintain for an easy run—you can produce enough body heat to offset the cold. The problem comes if you're exercising at a lower intensity, don't properly cover your skin, or get wet, which could leave you vulnerable to hypothermia or frostbite. You're most at risk for hypothermia when it's rainy or snowy out, or your skin is damp from sweat.

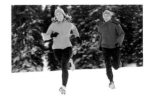

DID YOU KNOW?

Two strength-training sessions per week can improve your running. Add a third strength day to your routine in the 6 to 8 weeks before you start training for a race.

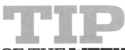

OF THE **WEEK**

Wearing worn-out or ill-fitting shoes is one of the most common causes of injury. Replace your shoes every 300 to 500 miles, and be sure to go to a specialty running shop, where you can get guidance on finding the shoe that offers the fit and support that your feet need.

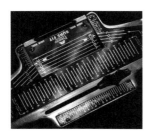

"Sport, like all life, is about taking risk."

—SIR ROGER BANNISTER,
first person to run a
sub 4–minute mile

MONDAY
ROUTE:

DISTANCE: TIME:

NOTES:

CROSS TRAINING:

TUESDAY
ROUTE:

DISTANCE: TIME:

NOTES:

CROSS TRAINING:

WEDNESDAY
ROUTE:

DISTANCE: TIME:

NOTES:

CROSS TRAINING:

THURSDAY
ROUTE:

DISTANCE: TIME:

NOTES:

CROSS TRAINING:

FRIDAY
ROUTE:

DISTANCE: TIME:

NOTES:

CROSS TRAINING:

SATURDAY

ROUTE:

DISTANCE: TIME:

NOTES:

CROSS TRAINING:

SUNDAY

ROUTE:

DISTANCE: TIME:

NOTES:

CROSS TRAINING:

NOTES

WEEKLY TOTAL

TOTAL MILEAGE TO DATE

TRAINING

TIGHT HAMSTRINGS?

The muscle groups at the backs of the legs—the hamstrings and calf muscles—are the best muscles for runners to stretch. Hamstring and hip-flexor flexibility seem to improve knee function, and calf flexibility may keep the Achilles tendon and plantar fascia healthy. Put one foot on an 8-inch step. Keep your toes pointed forward and knee slightly bent. Looking straight ahead, lean forward from your hips and pelvis while maintaining an arch in your lower back. Once you feel a stretch in the back of your thigh, hold the position for 15 to 30 seconds. Repeat on the other side.

DID YOU KNOW?

It's possible to overtrain—getting too little rest-whether you're logging 80 miles a week or 18. Early signs of overtraining include loss of energy and frequent fatigue. Your legs also might feel heavy and tired, even after a day off. Anxiety and irritability are other indicators. And at the extreme—but not uncommon—end, a runner who blasts through all the warning signals may wind up sick or even depressed.

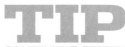

OF THE **WEEK**

If running becomes too complicated for you, forget your training plans for a day and put on a pair of running shoes. Then put one foot in front of the other. Simple? You bet. You'll be surprised at the result.

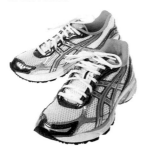

"I've always loved running . . . it was something you could do by yourself, and under your own power. You could go in any direction, fast or slow as you wanted, fighting the wind if you felt like it, seeking out new sights just on the strength of your feet and the courage of your lungs."

—JESSE OWENS,
Olympic 4-time gold medalist in 100 m dash, long jump, 200 m dash, and 400 m relay
(Berlin 1936)

MONDAY
ROUTE:

DISTANCE: TIME:

NOTES:

CROSS TRAINING:

TUESDAY
ROUTE:

DISTANCE: TIME:

NOTES:

CROSS TRAINING:

WEDNESDAY
ROUTE:

DISTANCE: TIME:

NOTES:

CROSS TRAINING:

THURSDAY
ROUTE:

DISTANCE: TIME:

NOTES:

CROSS TRAINING:

FRIDAY
ROUTE:

DISTANCE: TIME:

NOTES:

CROSS TRAINING:

SATURDAY

ROUTE:

DISTANCE: TIME:

NOTES:

CROSS TRAINING:

SUNDAY

ROUTE:

DISTANCE: TIME:

NOTES:

CROSS TRAINING:

NOTES

WEEKLY TOTAL

TOTAL MILEAGE TO DATE

NUTRITION

GOOD CARBS

Some carbohydrates are better than others. Remember that fresh fruits such as berries, melons, peaches, plums, and nectarines are loaded with carbohydrates—about 15 grams for every tennis ball–sized serving—and packed with vitamins and antioxidants. That's good stuff for runners.

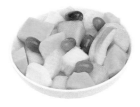

DID YOU KNOW?

The rest days you take are just as important as the miles you run. The body needs time to adapt to training changes and jumps in mileage or intensity. Muscles and joints need recovery time so they can handle more training demands. If you rush that process, you could break down rather than build up your body.

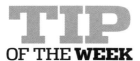

OF THE **WEEK**

A neuroma is an enlarged nerve, and it most frequently occurs in the interspace between the third and fourth toes. Though neuromas aren't visible, they can cause toe cramps or a more general pain in the ball of the foot. Hill running, which puts abnormal pressure on the ball of the foot, is a common cause of neuromas, so stick to the flats until the pain subsides. Your shoes might also be too tight in the toebox. Remove the insert, stand on it, and take a close look: If any portion of your foot is hanging over the insert, your shoes are too small.

"When you have the enthusiasm and the passion, you end up figuring out how to excel."

—DEENA KASTOR,
marathoner, Olympic bronze medalist (Athens 2004)

MONDAY
ROUTE:

DISTANCE: TIME:

NOTES:

CROSS TRAINING:

TUESDAY
ROUTE:

DISTANCE: TIME:

NOTES:

CROSS TRAINING:

WEDNESDAY
ROUTE:

DISTANCE: TIME:

NOTES:

CROSS TRAINING:

THURSDAY
ROUTE:

DISTANCE: TIME:

NOTES:

CROSS TRAINING:

FRIDAY
ROUTE:

DISTANCE: TIME:

NOTES:

CROSS TRAINING:

SATURDAY

ROUTE:

DISTANCE: TIME:

NOTES:

CROSS TRAINING:

SUNDAY

ROUTE:

DISTANCE: TIME:

NOTES:

CROSS TRAINING:

NOTES

WEEKLY TOTAL

TOTAL MILEAGE TO DATE

TRAINING

REST UP

Recent injuries? Take it easier. If you always seem to get injured just when you're getting really fit, it means you haven't let yourself fully adapt to your new training schedule. Back off by 10 to 20 percent of your weekly mileage for at least a month. If you still develop injuries at this lower level, back off again. It'll be frustrating, but not as frustrating as getting hurt and not being able to run at all.

DID YOU KNOW?

Use a sunscreen with an SPF of 30 or greater. It should be labeled "broad spectrum," which will protect you from UVA and UVB rays. Make sure that you apply enough sunscreen; the amount that could fill up a shot glass should cover your entire body before you go outside. Apply it 20 minutes before you go out so that it has time to be absorbed in the skin. If you're going on a long run, reapply the sunscreen once each hour.

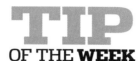

OF THE **WEEK**

Brazil nuts and Green tea can help buffer the harmful effects of the sun. Brazil nuts are nature's richest source of selenium, a mineral with antioxidant properties that may lessen skin damage due to ultraviolet radiation. Green tea is packed with polyphenols that may protect against UV-induced tumor development by reducing skin inflammation and DNA damage.

"I will always listen to my coaches. But first I listen to my body. If what they tell me suits my body, great. If my body doesn't feel good with what they say, then always my body comes first."

—HAILE GEBRSELASSIE,
Ethiopian, distance and marathon World record holder 2:03:59 (Berlin 2008)

MONDAY
ROUTE:

DISTANCE: TIME:

NOTES:

CROSS TRAINING:

TUESDAY
ROUTE:

DISTANCE: TIME:

NOTES:

CROSS TRAINING:

WEDNESDAY
ROUTE:

DISTANCE: TIME:

NOTES:

CROSS TRAINING:

THURSDAY
ROUTE:

DISTANCE: TIME:

NOTES:

CROSS TRAINING:

FRIDAY
ROUTE:

DISTANCE: TIME:

NOTES:

CROSS TRAINING:

SATURDAY

ROUTE:

DISTANCE: TIME:

NOTES:

CROSS TRAINING:

SUNDAY

ROUTE:

DISTANCE: TIME:

NOTES:

CROSS TRAINING:

NOTES

WEEKLY TOTAL

TOTAL MILEAGE TO DATE

NUTRITION

GOOD FATS

Your body won't run well on a totally fat-free diet. Runners need some fat each day to absorb the fat-soluble vitamins A, D, E, and K, which our bodies can't process by themselves. Research suggests that prostate-boosting lycopene and other anti-oxidants found in fruits and vegetables are absorbed better when combined with good fats.

DID YOU KNOW?

Hitting the Jacuzzi after a race might sound like a good idea, but you should avoid applying heat to sore muscles for 48 hours after a hard run or race. Instead, spend 6 to 8 minutes in a cold bath or swimming pool. Although it won't feel as good as a hot tub, the frigid water will combat inflammation and help you recover faster, so that you can start training in earnest for your next race.

TIP
OF THE **WEEK**

When you run, the soleus—one of the calf's two muscles—contracts in order to absorb the impact. A cold, inflexible muscle and dehydration magnify the stress on the muscle, which can lead to tightness. Drinking fluids an hour before you head out, starting each run with a 10-minute jog, and stretching and strengthening your calves will help keep them strong, loose, and pain free. Stretch after every workout. Place your hands on a wall and one foot in front of the other. Press the back heel to the ground, then bend the back knee slightly to target the soleus. Fatigue can also lead to tight calves, so build up miles gradually and take rest days.

"The miracle isn't that I finished. The miracle is that I had the courage to start."

—JOHN BINGHAM, marathoner and author; known as "The Penguin"

MONDAY
ROUTE:

DISTANCE: TIME:

NOTES:

CROSS TRAINING:

TUESDAY
ROUTE:

DISTANCE: TIME:

NOTES:

CROSS TRAINING:

WEDNESDAY
ROUTE:

DISTANCE: TIME:

NOTES:

CROSS TRAINING:

THURSDAY
ROUTE:

DISTANCE: TIME:

NOTES:

CROSS TRAINING:

FRIDAY
ROUTE:

DISTANCE: TIME:

NOTES:

CROSS TRAINING:

SATURDAY
ROUTE:

DISTANCE: TIME:

NOTES:

CROSS TRAINING:

SUNDAY
ROUTE:

DISTANCE: TIME:

NOTES:

CROSS TRAINING:

NOTES

WEEKLY TOTAL

TOTAL MILEAGE TO DATE

TRAINING

SEARCH YOUR SCHEDULE

If your schedule is jam-packed and you feel like you can't spare any time to run, try to find just 30 minutes on your calendar that you can set aside to exercise. Set the alarm 30 minutes early, run at the school while waiting for the kids to finish practice, or even sneak in 20 minutes over your lunch break.

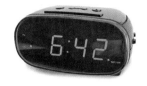

DID YOU KNOW?

A quick run keeps your muscles accustomed to the act of running, and after just 5 to 10 minutes, you start tapping into stored fat.

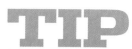

OF THE **WEEK**

Running on soft surfaces, like trails, dirt, and grass, can help reduce your risk of injury. If you're preparing for a road race, be sure to do some of your training on the roads.

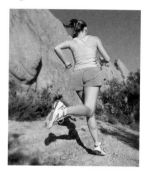

"Any runner who denies having fears, nerves, or some kind of disposition is a bad athlete, or a liar."

—GORDON PIRIE, English cross-country and distance runner, Olympic 5,000 m silver medalist (Melbourne 1956)

MONDAY
ROUTE:

DISTANCE: TIME:

NOTES:

CROSS TRAINING:

TUESDAY
ROUTE:

DISTANCE: TIME:

NOTES:

CROSS TRAINING:

WEDNESDAY
ROUTE:

DISTANCE: TIME:

NOTES:

CROSS TRAINING:

THURSDAY
ROUTE:

DISTANCE: TIME:

NOTES:

CROSS TRAINING:

FRIDAY
ROUTE:

DISTANCE: TIME:

NOTES:

CROSS TRAINING:

SATURDAY

ROUTE:

DISTANCE: TIME:

NOTES:

CROSS TRAINING:

SUNDAY

ROUTE:

DISTANCE: TIME:

NOTES:

CROSS TRAINING:

NOTES

WEEKLY TOTAL

TOTAL MILEAGE TO DATE

NUTRITION

PRERUN SNACKS

To curb prerun hunger, eat high-carb, low-fiber foods that are easy to digest and that provide fast energy 30 to 60 minutes before running. Eat some protein and fat to steady your blood sugar during a long run, but consume sparingly. Have a piece of fruit paired with cottage cheese. Other options: fig cookies or half a bagel with nut butter and jam.

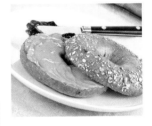

DID YOU KNOW?

Everyone gets nervous before a race. Try using visualization and "see" the race beforehand to settle down. Anticipate the steps involved— waking up, driving to the site, running the race, crossing the finish line, and then returning home. Stomach butter- flies and fears will decrease once you have gone through the motions in your mind.

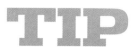

OF THE **WEEK**

If you're dealing with plantar fasciitis—irritation of the tissue that connects the big toe and forefoot with the heel, forming the lining of the arch—you may feel a sharp pain first thing in the morning because the plantar fascia shortens during the night, while you're asleep. When you get out of bed in the morning and start walking around, the band along the bottom of your foot stretches and pulls on your heel. When it pulls too hard, pain results. To ease the pain, submerge your foot in ice water for 10 minutes several times a day. Wear a heel cup or heel cushion in both running and regular shoes. Give your foot about 4 to 6 weeks without running to heal completely.

"Even if you're inches away from the finish, never take success for granted."

—DEAN KARNAZES, author, ultramarathoner, and finisher of 50 marathons in 50 states in 50 days

MONDAY
ROUTE:

DISTANCE: TIME:

NOTES:

CROSS TRAINING:

TUESDAY
ROUTE:

DISTANCE: TIME:

NOTES:

CROSS TRAINING:

WEDNESDAY
ROUTE:

DISTANCE: TIME:

NOTES:

CROSS TRAINING:

THURSDAY
ROUTE:

DISTANCE: TIME:

NOTES:

CROSS TRAINING:

FRIDAY
ROUTE:

DISTANCE: TIME:

NOTES:

CROSS TRAINING:

SATURDAY

ROUTE:

DISTANCE: TIME:

NOTES:

CROSS TRAINING:

SUNDAY

ROUTE:

DISTANCE: TIME:

NOTES:

CROSS TRAINING:

NOTES

WEEKLY TOTAL

TOTAL MILEAGE TO DATE

TRAINING

HEALTHY HEELS

Heel whip is a condition that causes your ankle-bone to get beat up by the opposite heel due to the excessive rotational motion of your foot. Instead of your foot traveling in a forward plane, it makes an arc, causing your heel to nick your anklebone. Push off through your big toe, not your pinkie toe, so that your foot swings cleanly forward, and you'll be less likely to hit your ankle.

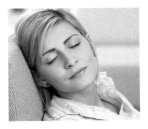

DID YOU KNOW?

Research shows that short naps decrease fatigue and improve alertness and cognitive performance—and you need only 10 minutes of shut-eye to reap the benefits. In fact, sleeping for 10 minutes is superior to taking a 20- or 30-minute snooze because you're less likely to be groggy or confused upon waking up.

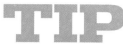

OF THE **WEEK**

Need a little guidance when deciding whether to run on the trail? **It's okay** to run on a trail if you've struggled with runner's knee, iliotibial band syndrome (ITBS), shin splints, or any injury aggravated by impact. Just be wary of technical trails that cause your feet to land at an angle. **It's not okay** to run on a trail if you've had an ankle sprain. The ligaments of that joint never recover 100 percent. That increases your risk of a repeat sprain on soft, uneven surfaces.

"I always try to impress upon the kids to be grateful and to learn from the hard times they have in running because it is such a metaphor for life. We always hear this, but it is amazing how true it is and how much high school running can shape someone for the rest of their life."

—DATHAN RITZENHEIN,
cross-country, distance, and marathon runner, Olympian in 10,000 m (Athens 2004)

MONDAY
ROUTE:

DISTANCE: TIME:

NOTES:

CROSS TRAINING:

TUESDAY
ROUTE:

DISTANCE: TIME:

NOTES:

CROSS TRAINING:

WEDNESDAY
ROUTE:

DISTANCE: TIME:

NOTES:

CROSS TRAINING:

THURSDAY
ROUTE:

DISTANCE: TIME:

NOTES:

CROSS TRAINING:

FRIDAY
ROUTE:

DISTANCE: TIME:

NOTES:

CROSS TRAINING:

SATURDAY

ROUTE:

DISTANCE: TIME:

NOTES:

CROSS TRAINING:

SUNDAY

ROUTE:

DISTANCE: TIME:

NOTES:

CROSS TRAINING:

NOTES

WEEKLY TOTAL

TOTAL MILEAGE TO DATE

NUTRITION

THE BEST CARBS

Slow-burning carbs are high in fiber and are slowly digested. They keep your blood sugar steady, provide long-lasting energy, and should be a staple of your diet. Where can you find them? In oatmeal and other whole grains, beans, lentils, fruits, and vegetables. Fast-burning carbs are digested quickly, are low in fiber, and have a greater effect on your blood sugar. They provide a quick hit of energy that's useful to runners right before working out, but you should eat them in moderation. Where can you find them? In pasta, white rice, white flour, potatoes, and cornflakes.

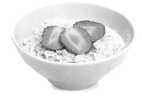

DID YOU KNOW?

People who run more than 35 miles a week are 54 percent less likely to suffer age-related vision loss than those who cover 10 miles a week.

TIP
OF THE WEEK

Whether running on flat terrain or up hills, keep your eyes directly ahead of you, not down at your feet. You're less likely to slouch and trip and you'll move up the hill more easily.

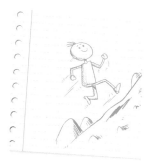

"Hills are speedwork in disguise."

—FRANK SHORTER,
marathoner, Olympic gold (Munich 1972) and silver (Montreal 1976) medalist

MONDAY
ROUTE:

DISTANCE: TIME:

NOTES:

CROSS TRAINING:

TUESDAY
ROUTE:

DISTANCE: TIME:

NOTES:

CROSS TRAINING:

WEDNESDAY
ROUTE:

DISTANCE: TIME:

NOTES:

CROSS TRAINING:

THURSDAY
ROUTE:

DISTANCE: TIME:

NOTES:

CROSS TRAINING:

FRIDAY
ROUTE:

DISTANCE: TIME:

NOTES:

CROSS TRAINING:

SATURDAY

ROUTE:

DISTANCE: TIME:

NOTES:

CROSS TRAINING:

SUNDAY

ROUTE:

DISTANCE: TIME:

NOTES:

CROSS TRAINING:

NOTES

WEEKLY TOTAL

TOTAL MILEAGE TO DATE

TRAINING

TREADMILL TRAINING

If you can't go outside to train on hills, try this: Warm up on a treadmill at no incline. Then increase the incline by two levels every 2 minutes until you hit level 12. (Run 1 to 2 minutes slower than your normal training pace while you do this.) Descend in the same manner, decreasing by two levels every 2 minutes.

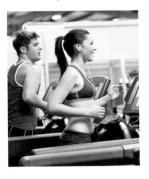

DID YOU KNOW?

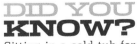

Sitting in a cold tub for 10 to 20 minutes after a hard workout helps reduce inflammation.

TIP
OF THE **WEEK**

The quinine in 8 ounces of tonic water may help ward off or reduce the severity of night leg cramps. Try drinking the bubbly stuff before bedtime. (Lime wedge optional.)

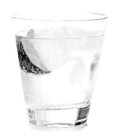

"You've got to look at what your weaknesses are and then work on them . . . If you're not so good on hills, you've got to run a lot of hills. The goal has to be to perfect the things that you're not as good at yet."

—LYNN JENNINGS,
cross-country, track, and middle distance runner, Olympic 10,000 m bronze medalist (Barcelona 1992); American record holder for 10,000 m

MONDAY
ROUTE:

DISTANCE: TIME:

NOTES:

CROSS TRAINING:

TUESDAY
ROUTE:

DISTANCE: TIME:

NOTES:

CROSS TRAINING:

WEDNESDAY
ROUTE:

DISTANCE: TIME:

NOTES:

CROSS TRAINING:

THURSDAY
ROUTE:

DISTANCE: TIME:

NOTES:

CROSS TRAINING:

FRIDAY
ROUTE:

DISTANCE: TIME:

NOTES:

CROSS TRAINING:

SATURDAY

ROUTE:

DISTANCE: TIME:

NOTES:

CROSS TRAINING:

SUNDAY

ROUTE:

DISTANCE: TIME:

NOTES:

CROSS TRAINING:

NOTES

WEEKLY TOTAL

TOTAL MILEAGE TO DATE

NUTRITION

CONSCIOUS INDULGENCES

Indulgences are as necessary as training. If the ice cream cake is for a really special occasion, have a slice, then make a compromise later in the day. Save the nuts and fruit you brought for a snack for tomorrow. If your office is constantly stacked with treats, move them into the fridge and put a sign on the front that simply says, "Goodies Inside!" It's easier to resist treats you can't see.

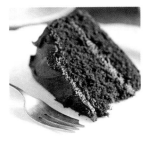

DID YOU KNOW?

Men who burn at least 3,000 calories per week (equal to about 5 hours of running) are 83 percent less likely to have severe erectile dysfunction.

TIP
OF THE **WEEK**

If you're out on a run and your shoulders begin to feel tight, unclench your fists. Keep your hands and wrists loose. Loose hands help your whole body stay relaxed.

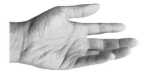

"The long run is what puts the tiger in the cat."

—BILL SQUIRES, coach of Alberto Salazar and other elite marathoners

MONDAY
ROUTE:

DISTANCE: TIME:

NOTES:

CROSS TRAINING:

TUESDAY
ROUTE:

DISTANCE: TIME:

NOTES:

CROSS TRAINING:

WEDNESDAY
ROUTE:

DISTANCE: TIME:

NOTES:

CROSS TRAINING:

THURSDAY
ROUTE:

DISTANCE: TIME:

NOTES:

CROSS TRAINING:

FRIDAY
ROUTE:

DISTANCE: TIME:

NOTES:

CROSS TRAINING:

SATURDAY

ROUTE:

DISTANCE: TIME:

NOTES:

CROSS TRAINING:

SUNDAY

ROUTE:

DISTANCE: TIME:

NOTES:

CROSS TRAINING:

NOTES

WEEKLY TOTAL

TOTAL MILEAGE TO DATE

TRAINING

7-MINUTE SECRET

Seven minutes of exercise a day—that's all you need to build strength. Do these exercises: Reverse lunges, single-leg hops, single-leg reach (similar to the Warrior III yoga pose), planks with alternate leg lift, and a squat with both hands up (called a Y-squat). For most exercises, do 8 reps (or 8 on each side).

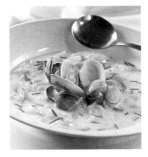

DID YOU KNOW?

Dishes like carb-rich seafood chowder can fortify your defenses. Carbs protect weak immune cells and the zinc in seafood supports immune health.

TIP
OF THE **WEEK**

Before giving up your gym membership, ask for a customized plan. As a runner, you're probably using only a portion of the gym and don't need access to that 7 a.m. kickboxing class. Tell the owner what you do use: free weights, a few exercise machines, and oh yeah, the treadmill. If he or she cannot reduce your fee by making it based on sessions used, then look for a niche gym that tailors programs to clients' needs.

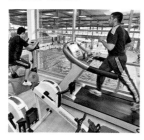

"You have to forget your last marathon before you try another. Your mind can't know what's coming."

—FRANK SHORTER,
marathoner, Olympic gold (Munich 1972) and silver (Montreal 1976) medalist

MONDAY
ROUTE:

DISTANCE: TIME:

NOTES:

CROSS TRAINING:

TUESDAY
ROUTE:

DISTANCE: TIME:

NOTES:

CROSS TRAINING:

WEDNESDAY
ROUTE:

DISTANCE: TIME:

NOTES:

CROSS TRAINING:

THURSDAY
ROUTE:

DISTANCE: TIME:

NOTES:

CROSS TRAINING:

FRIDAY
ROUTE:

DISTANCE: TIME:

NOTES:

CROSS TRAINING:

SATURDAY

ROUTE:

DISTANCE: TIME:

NOTES:

CROSS TRAINING:

SUNDAY

ROUTE:

DISTANCE: TIME:

NOTES:

CROSS TRAINING:

NOTES

WEEKLY TOTAL

TOTAL MILEAGE TO DATE

TRAINING

TOUGH WORKOUT

Used for years by the University of Michigan's men's distance team, this workout should not be undertaken lightly. Run a mile. Run a 400 on a nearby track. Run a mile on the road. Run an 800. Run another mile on the road. Run a 1200. Your only rest is a 200-meter jog between the road and the track.

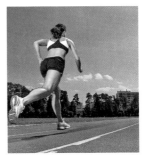

DID YOU KNOW?

People who exercise for an hour a day are 18 percent less likely to suffer upper respiratory tract infections than those who are inactive, according to a study from Sweden. Moderate activity boosts immunity.

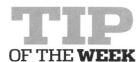

OF THE **WEEK**

Have work or family commitments cut into your training? Then remember to cut back on your eating. If you're not running as much, you don't need as much food to fuel your efforts. Failure to do so may result in tighter shorts.

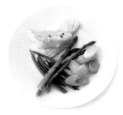

"The gun goes off and everything changes . . . the world changes . . . and nothing else really matters."

—PATTISUE PLUMER,
Olympian in the 1500 m (Seoul 1988) and 1500 m and 3000 m (Barcelona 1992); Goodwill Games gold and bronze medalist (1990)

MONDAY
ROUTE:

DISTANCE: TIME:

NOTES:

CROSS TRAINING:

TUESDAY
ROUTE:

DISTANCE: TIME:

NOTES:

CROSS TRAINING:

WEDNESDAY
ROUTE:

DISTANCE: TIME:

NOTES:

CROSS TRAINING:

THURSDAY
ROUTE:

DISTANCE: TIME:

NOTES:

CROSS TRAINING:

FRIDAY
ROUTE:

DISTANCE: TIME:

NOTES:

CROSS TRAINING:

SATURDAY

ROUTE:

DISTANCE: TIME:

NOTES:

CROSS TRAINING:

SUNDAY

ROUTE:

DISTANCE: TIME:

NOTES:

CROSS TRAINING:

NOTES

WEEKLY TOTAL

TOTAL MILEAGE TO DATE

NUTRITION

SKIP THE BOOZE

Skip the celebratory cocktails the night before your race. It's tempting to ease the nervousness with a drink, but if you normally avoid alcohol, don't drink the night before or the day of the marathon. However, if you're accustomed to drinking alcohol, one drink the night before a race won't hamper your running.

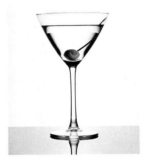

DID YOU KNOW?

Joan Benoit Samuelson, winner of the 1984 Olympic marathon, broke her US 50-to-54 mark with a 2:47:50 at the October 2010 Chicago Marathon.

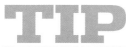

OF THE **WEEK**

Implement the buddy system if your training is lagging. You may get more from your workout when you run with other people. Don't know of anyone to run with? Check out your local running club. A running club is a great place to find other runners who run your pace. Running clubs include runners at every level. Visit www.rrca.org /find-a-running-club to find a club in your area.

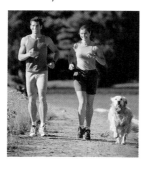

"Wisely and slow; they stumble that run fast."

—WILLIAM SHAKESPEARE,
Romeo and Juliet

MONDAY
ROUTE:

DISTANCE: TIME:

NOTES:

CROSS TRAINING:

TUESDAY
ROUTE:

DISTANCE: TIME:

NOTES:

CROSS TRAINING:

WEDNESDAY
ROUTE:

DISTANCE: TIME:

NOTES:

CROSS TRAINING:

THURSDAY
ROUTE:

DISTANCE: TIME:

NOTES:

CROSS TRAINING:

FRIDAY
ROUTE:

DISTANCE: TIME:

NOTES:

CROSS TRAINING:

SATURDAY

ROUTE:

DISTANCE: TIME:

NOTES:

CROSS TRAINING:

SUNDAY

ROUTE:

DISTANCE: TIME:

NOTES:

CROSS TRAINING:

NOTES

WEEKLY TOTAL

TOTAL MILEAGE TO DATE

TRAINING

TRY A PLANK!

Planks, done correctly, can give you a supersolid core. Side planks, which are even more effective, hit the obliques, transversus abdominis, lower back, hips, and glutes. Lie on your right side, supporting your upper body on your right forearm, with your left arm at your left side. Lift your hips and, keeping your body weight supported on your forearm and the side of your right foot, extend your left arm above your shoulder. Hold this position for 10 to 30 seconds. Switch sides and repeat. Keep your hips up; don't let them sag.

DID YOU KNOW?

One big mistake runners make when icing an injury is taking the cold pack off too soon. If you ice for less than 10 minutes, you'll cool your skin, but there will be minimal effect on the underlying muscle tissue. In general, 15 to 20 minutes is ideal.

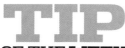

OF THE **WEEK**

If your doctor has forbidden you from hitting the road or track until an injury heals but you don't want to lose running-specific fitness, hop in the pool for deep-water running sessions. Wear a flotation belt to improve your buoyancy and run as you normally would, keeping your feet off the bottom of the pool, of course. You can maintain your fitness for as long as 6 weeks on pool running alone.

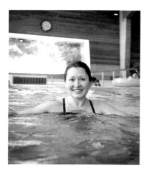

"Life is short . . . running makes it longer."

—JAMES EDWARD, BARON HANSON, amateur runner and English businessman

MONDAY
ROUTE:

DISTANCE:　　　　　　　　TIME:

NOTES:

CROSS TRAINING:

TUESDAY
ROUTE:

DISTANCE:　　　　　　　　TIME:

NOTES:

CROSS TRAINING:

WEDNESDAY
ROUTE:

DISTANCE:　　　　　　　　TIME:

NOTES:

CROSS TRAINING:

THURSDAY
ROUTE:

DISTANCE:　　　　　　　　TIME:

NOTES:

CROSS TRAINING:

FRIDAY
ROUTE:

DISTANCE:　　　　　　　　TIME:

NOTES:

CROSS TRAINING:

SATURDAY

ROUTE:

DISTANCE: TIME:

NOTES:

CROSS TRAINING:

SUNDAY

ROUTE:

DISTANCE: TIME:

NOTES:

CROSS TRAINING:

NOTES

WEEKLY TOTAL

TOTAL MILEAGE TO DATE

TRAINING

INCREASE YOUR SPEED

If you want to increase speed for a 5-K or a 10-K, do one speed session a week. If you want to run a faster marathon, run mile repeats on weekends when you're not doing a long run. Short but fast workouts help maintain the function of your spinal cord's motor nerve cells, the ones that control fast running. Without high-quality speedwork, these cells deteriorate as you get older, slowing you down. And researchers at the Institute for Olympic Sports in Finland found that for average runners, there is much to be gained from running sprint intervals of 50 to 200 meters once a week.

DID YOU KNOW?

At mile 13 of the Big Sur International Marathon in California, a pianist in a tuxedo plays "Chariots of Fire."

TIP
OF THE **WEEK**

Because speedwork is an intense workout, it should be spaced out from long runs by at least 2 days. You need to recover from mile repeats before tackling a 15-miler, and vice versa. Do weekly speed sessions for the 6 to 10 weeks leading up to a race. Any more than that and the results will start to plateau. Some form of fast running, like short sprints, should be part of your running workout year-round.

"It's very hard in the beginning to understand that the whole idea is not to beat the other runners. Eventually you learn that the competition is against the little voice inside you that wants you to quit."

—GEORGE SHEEHAN, MD,
track and distance runner, author, and former medical editor for *Runner's World*

MONDAY
ROUTE:

DISTANCE: TIME:

NOTES:

CROSS TRAINING:

TUESDAY
ROUTE:

DISTANCE: TIME:

NOTES:

CROSS TRAINING:

WEDNESDAY
ROUTE:

DISTANCE: TIME:

NOTES:

CROSS TRAINING:

THURSDAY
ROUTE:

DISTANCE: TIME:

NOTES:

CROSS TRAINING:

FRIDAY
ROUTE:

DISTANCE: TIME:

NOTES:

CROSS TRAINING:

SATURDAY

ROUTE:

DISTANCE: TIME:

NOTES:

CROSS TRAINING:

SUNDAY

ROUTE:

DISTANCE: TIME:

NOTES:

CROSS TRAINING:

NOTES

WEEKLY TOTAL

TOTAL MILEAGE TO DATE

NUTRITION

LIGHT LUNCH

The key to a lunch that won't ruin your lunch run is to keep it light, keep it low in fiber, and time it right. Around 10 a.m., eat one energy bar or a large handful of pretzel nuggets and have 16 ounces of sports drink. Afterward, enjoy half of a turkey wrap with light mayo.

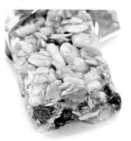

DID YOU KNOW?

Studies suggest that athletes perform best in the late afternoon—when most of us are still at work or on car pool duty. Fortunately, research also shows that we can train our bodies to run well at any time of day simply by exercising regularly at that time.

TIP
OF THE **WEEK**

If you want to get the most out of cross training, keep it intense. Adding a few spurts of effort on your bike or in the pool will raise your heart rate and work different muscle groups.

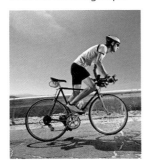

"To truly enjoy running, test yourself. If you win, fine. If you lose, this gives you the incentive to keep trying. You have to train a bit harder, and you have to come back again and again. That is the joy."

—RON CLARKE, Australian distance runner; Olympic 10,000 m bronze medalist (Tokyo 1964)

MONDAY
ROUTE:

DISTANCE: TIME:

NOTES:

CROSS TRAINING:

TUESDAY
ROUTE:

DISTANCE: TIME:

NOTES:

CROSS TRAINING:

WEDNESDAY
ROUTE:

DISTANCE: TIME:

NOTES:

CROSS TRAINING:

THURSDAY
ROUTE:

DISTANCE: TIME:

NOTES:

CROSS TRAINING:

FRIDAY
ROUTE:

DISTANCE: TIME:

NOTES:

CROSS TRAINING:

SATURDAY
ROUTE:

DISTANCE: TIME:

NOTES:

CROSS TRAINING:

SUNDAY
ROUTE:

DISTANCE: TIME:

NOTES:

CROSS TRAINING:

NOTES

WEEKLY TOTAL

TOTAL MILEAGE TO DATE

TRAINING

WARMUP WISDOM

The speed of your warmup should reflect your intended race pace and your race distance. If you're racing a 5-K, a relatively short distance compared to a half- or full marathon, your pace will be relatively fast. As such, you'll need to rev up your muscles beforehand. Some short, fast intervals at just above race pace can prepare you to sustain that pace on the racecourse.

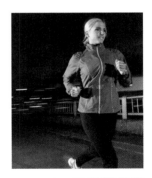

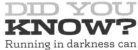

DID YOU KNOW?

Running in darkness can make you *feel* faster.

TIP
OF THE **WEEK**

Never increase your weekly mileage by more than 10 percent. The vast majority of injuries suffered by runners are the result of overuse. So if you've been doing 25 miles a week for a while and want to run more, add a maximum of 2.5 miles next week.

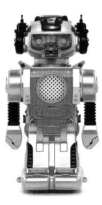

"We would like to be robots and turn the knob to our goal pace and just go, but we're human."

—GREG MCMILLAN,
marathoner, coach, and owner of McMillan Running Company

MONDAY
ROUTE:

DISTANCE: TIME:

NOTES:

CROSS TRAINING:

TUESDAY
ROUTE:

DISTANCE: TIME:

NOTES:

CROSS TRAINING:

WEDNESDAY
ROUTE:

DISTANCE: TIME:

NOTES:

CROSS TRAINING:

THURSDAY
ROUTE:

DISTANCE: TIME:

NOTES:

CROSS TRAINING:

FRIDAY
ROUTE:

DISTANCE: TIME:

NOTES:

CROSS TRAINING:

SATURDAY

ROUTE:

DISTANCE: TIME:

NOTES:

CROSS TRAINING:

SUNDAY

ROUTE:

DISTANCE: TIME:

NOTES:

CROSS TRAINING:

NOTES

WEEKLY TOTAL

TOTAL MILEAGE TO DATE

TRAINING

RUNNING FOR RUNNING'S SAKE

Every once in a while, leave all of your running toys at home and simply run so that it feels good. The simple act of striding along without a watch or a heart rate monitor telling you how you're doing will help you remember why you started lacing 'em up in the first place.

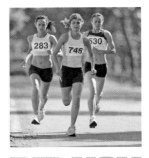

DID YOU KNOW?

There are two women-only US marathons (Leading Ladies' Marathon, South Dakota; Nike Women's Marathon, California).

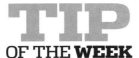

OF THE **WEEK**

Slow miles burn almost as many calories as fast miles. Fast or slow, each mile you run burns approximately 100 calories. That keeps your weight down, which in turn can help you run faster.

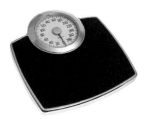

"Everybody and their mother knows you don't train hard on Friday, the day before a race. But a lot of runners will overtrain on Thursday if left on their own. Thursday is the most dangerous day of the week."

—MARTY STERN, legendary NCAA coach

MONDAY
ROUTE:

DISTANCE: TIME:

NOTES:

CROSS TRAINING:

TUESDAY
ROUTE:

DISTANCE: TIME:

NOTES:

CROSS TRAINING:

WEDNESDAY
ROUTE:

DISTANCE: TIME:

NOTES:

CROSS TRAINING:

THURSDAY
ROUTE:

DISTANCE: TIME:

NOTES:

CROSS TRAINING:

FRIDAY
ROUTE:

DISTANCE: TIME:

NOTES:

CROSS TRAINING:

SATURDAY

ROUTE:

DISTANCE: TIME:

NOTES:

CROSS TRAINING:

SUNDAY

ROUTE:

DISTANCE: TIME:

NOTES:

CROSS TRAINING:

NOTES

WEEKLY TOTAL

TOTAL MILEAGE TO DATE

TRAINING

LACING UP

Do you have a hard time keeping your running shoelaces tied? Consider using flat laces, which tend to hold knots better than round laces do. Your shoes may not feel as snug with flat laces, but you're less likely to have to stop mid-run to retie your shoes with them.

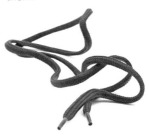

DID YOU KNOW?

The daily recommendation of eyesight-sharpening vitamin A can be found in one sweet potato.

TIP
OF THE **WEEK**

Here's a handy way to select the right amount of clothing to wear while running during cold weather: If the temperature is between 60°F and 41°F, wear one layer on both your upper and lower body. If it's between 40°F and 11°F, wear two upper-body layers and one on your lower body. Between 9°F and –20°F, wear three upper-body layers and two on your lower body. If it's colder than –20°F, curl up with a good book.

"The difference . . . is that you meet your goal unless something prevents it. Hot, tired, and a little out of it doesn't cut it; injury, dizziness, something inexplicably wrong, yes. Half of this distance running thing is being tough, isn't it?"

—MARK BITTMAN, runner, chef, author, and *New York Times* columnist

MONDAY
ROUTE:

DISTANCE: TIME:

NOTES:

CROSS TRAINING:

TUESDAY
ROUTE:

DISTANCE: TIME:

NOTES:

CROSS TRAINING:

WEDNESDAY
ROUTE:

DISTANCE: TIME:

NOTES:

CROSS TRAINING:

THURSDAY
ROUTE:

DISTANCE: TIME:

NOTES:

CROSS TRAINING:

FRIDAY
ROUTE:

DISTANCE: TIME:

NOTES:

CROSS TRAINING:

SATURDAY

ROUTE:

DISTANCE: TIME:

NOTES:

CROSS TRAINING:

SUNDAY

ROUTE:

DISTANCE: TIME:

NOTES:

CROSS TRAINING:

NOTES

WEEKLY TOTAL

TOTAL MILEAGE TO DATE

NUTRITION

FIBER UP

Slow your digestion and feel fuller throughout the day by having some fiber at every meal. Spreading out your fiber intake will also help you to avoid stomach discomfort during a run.

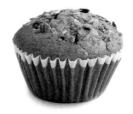

DID YOU KNOW?

Marathons have never been more popular. Approximately 518,000 people finished a marathon in 2011, according to RunningUSA.org. That's up 47 percent since 2000.

TIP
OF THE WEEK

Sure, running improves your mood, but a study conducted at the University of Helsinki shows that people who exercise in bright sunlight experience more relief from depression than people who exercise under indoor lighting. So remember what your mom told you: Go outside and play.

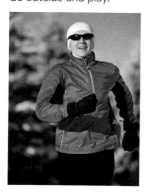

"You have to think that you can't quit. Your brain wants to quit, but you have to fight it. It has nothing to do with speed and everything to do with finishing."

—ABE WEINTRAUB, who completed 9 New York City Marathons while in his eighties

MONDAY
ROUTE:

DISTANCE: TIME:

NOTES:

CROSS TRAINING:

TUESDAY
ROUTE:

DISTANCE: TIME:

NOTES:

CROSS TRAINING:

WEDNESDAY
ROUTE:

DISTANCE: TIME:

NOTES:

CROSS TRAINING:

THURSDAY
ROUTE:

DISTANCE: TIME:

NOTES:

CROSS TRAINING:

FRIDAY
ROUTE:

DISTANCE: TIME:

NOTES:

CROSS TRAINING:

SATURDAY

ROUTE:

DISTANCE: TIME:

NOTES:

CROSS TRAINING:

SUNDAY

ROUTE:

DISTANCE: TIME:

NOTES:

CROSS TRAINING:

NOTES

WEEKLY TOTAL

TOTAL MILEAGE TO DATE

NUTRITION

SLOW FOOD

Eat slowly if you want to lose weight. It takes 20 minutes for your body to register that it's full, so it's easy to load up on extra calories if you're speed-eating. Take the time to savor each bite and watch the pounds melt away.

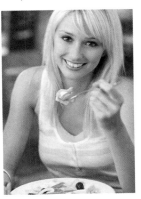

DID YOU KNOW?

If you're doing your running when the sun isn't shining, you could have low levels of vitamin D, a nutrient essential for calcium absorption.

TIP
OF THE **WEEK**

Now that you're keeping a written training journal, consider keeping a photo journal, too. Either you or your running buddy should grab your picture (on a cell phone camera) after a great run. Save it, print it, and keep it on your computer or in this journal so that you'll remember how you felt (or looked) for motivation on your blah days.

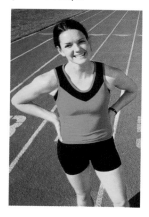

"Anyone can run 20 miles. It's the next 6 that count."

—BARRY MAGEE, New Zealander; marathon Olympic bronze medalist (Rome 1960)

MONDAY
ROUTE:

DISTANCE: TIME:

NOTES:

CROSS TRAINING:

TUESDAY
ROUTE:

DISTANCE: TIME:

NOTES:

CROSS TRAINING:

WEDNESDAY
ROUTE:

DISTANCE: TIME:

NOTES:

CROSS TRAINING:

THURSDAY
ROUTE:

DISTANCE: TIME:

NOTES:

CROSS TRAINING:

FRIDAY
ROUTE:

DISTANCE: TIME:

NOTES:

CROSS TRAINING:

SATURDAY

ROUTE:

DISTANCE: TIME:

NOTES:

CROSS TRAINING:

SUNDAY

ROUTE:

DISTANCE: TIME:

NOTES:

CROSS TRAINING:

NOTES

WEEKLY TOTAL

TOTAL MILEAGE TO DATE

NUTRITION

THE BEST RED MEAT

Don't be fooled into thinking that all red meat is high in fat. Sweet-tasting bison— or buffalo—is lower in saturated fat than conventional beef and is rich in protein: 5 ounces have almost one-third of most runners' daily needs. Many bison are raised on a grass diet, and as a result, studies show that they have higher levels of heart-healthy omega-3s than corn-fed beef. Plus, ranchers are banned from using hormones in any bison intended for food consumption. Use bison instead of ground beef in your cooking. WARNING: Bison is very lean, so it will cook—and overcook—faster than beef.

DID YOU KNOW?

A study in the *Journal of the American College of Nutrition* found that eating almond butter for 4 weeks reduced harmful LDL and raised beneficial HDL. So if you're sick of peanut butter, give it a try. Almond butter also packs more bone-building minerals like magnesium, calcium, and phosphorus, and more vitamin E than PB.

TIP
OF THE **WEEK**

Potassium is a mineral that works with sodium (also a mineral) to balance the fluid and electrolyte levels in your body. And since steady fluid levels help to regulate your heartbeat and prevent muscles from cramping, potassium is of particular importance to runners. No need to supplement, just eat fruits and veggies. Good sources of potassium include bananas, nectarines, baked potatoes, and carrots.

"It's the heart of that runner that God sees as great and the ability they have to run with a heart full of love for God, self, and others—not the speed of their legs."

—RYAN HALL, Olympic marathoner

MONDAY
ROUTE:

DISTANCE: TIME:

NOTES:

CROSS TRAINING:

TUESDAY
ROUTE:

DISTANCE: TIME:

NOTES:

CROSS TRAINING:

WEDNESDAY
ROUTE:

DISTANCE: TIME:

NOTES:

CROSS TRAINING:

THURSDAY
ROUTE:

DISTANCE: TIME:

NOTES:

CROSS TRAINING:

FRIDAY
ROUTE:

DISTANCE: TIME:

NOTES:

CROSS TRAINING:

SATURDAY
ROUTE:

DISTANCE: TIME:

NOTES:

CROSS TRAINING:

SUNDAY
ROUTE:

DISTANCE: TIME:

NOTES:

CROSS TRAINING:

NOTES

WEEKLY TOTAL

TOTAL MILEAGE TO DATE

TRAINING

HAPPY FEET

Specialty running stores can help you choose the best insoles for your feet and shoes. Insoles from these shops usually cost $20 to $40 and last about a year. Before you buy, press on the arch of the insert. If it collapses, it's not supportive enough. Also, don't buy half-insoles that just go under your heel. You push off the ball of your foot, and that's when your foot pronates and collapses inward, so the insole needs to go under your entire foot. If you find insoles that help—but not 100 percent—take them to a podiatrist, who can customize them. It's cheaper ($75 to $100) than a prescription orthotic and may work just as well.

DID YOU KNOW?

Runners need to eat 0.45 to 0.72 grams of protein per pound of body weight each day to speed muscle growth and rebuild fibers stressed by workouts. That's 75 to 120 grams of protein for a 165-pound runner.

TIP
OF THE **WEEK**

Think about utilizing a personal trainer for your cross-training workouts. The benefits are more psychological than physical: You'll get another person's full and complete attention. He or she will focus specifically and intently on what you're doing, how you're doing it, how often you're doing it, how many more times you should do it, and when you need a break from doing it to go get a drink of water.

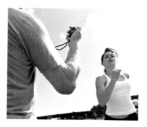

"You were running so well. Who has held you back from following the truth?"

—GALATIANS 5:7
(Paul of Tarsus)

MONDAY
ROUTE:

DISTANCE: TIME:

NOTES:

CROSS TRAINING:

TUESDAY
ROUTE:

DISTANCE: TIME:

NOTES:

CROSS TRAINING:

WEDNESDAY
ROUTE:

DISTANCE: TIME:

NOTES:

CROSS TRAINING:

THURSDAY
ROUTE:

DISTANCE: TIME:

NOTES:

CROSS TRAINING:

FRIDAY
ROUTE:

DISTANCE: TIME:

NOTES:

CROSS TRAINING:

SATURDAY

ROUTE:

DISTANCE: TIME:

NOTES:

CROSS TRAINING:

SUNDAY

ROUTE:

DISTANCE: TIME:

NOTES:

CROSS TRAINING:

NOTES

WEEKLY TOTAL

TOTAL MILEAGE TO DATE

NUTRITION

THE GREAT PUMPKIN

Pumpkin is not just for Halloween anymore. Use it in soups, dips, breads, and yes, desserts. For recipe suggestions, go to http:// recipes.runnersworld.com /RecipeFinder.aspx.

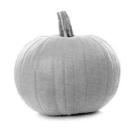

DID YOU KNOW?

If your knees crack, you're not alone. Crepitus, the medical term, happens when cartilage, the connective tissue between bones, starts to age. Over time, it becomes gray and old and doesn't regenerate; most people older than age 30 have some mild crepitus. Weak quads or a tight IT band can pull the kneecaps out of alignment and exacerbate the wear and tear.

TIP
OF THE **WEEK**

If your legs are still moving while you're sleeping, you may have skimped on a post-run meal. When you work hard and sweat, you excrete a lot of sodium and calcium, two electrolytes that are responsible for muscle relaxation. Iron deficiency, especially in women, can also contribute. Get up and head to the kitchen for a glass of milk and some pretzels. Avoid future leg-twitching problems and make sure to include dairy, salt, and iron, found in lean red meat and spinach, in your meals after a run.

"Life is often compared to a marathon, but I think it is more like being a sprinter; long stretches of hard work punctuated by brief moments in which we are given the opportunity to perform at our best."

—MICHAEL JOHNSON,
Olympic sprinter and
gold medalist (Barcelona 1992,
Atlanta 1996, and Sydney 2000)

MONDAY
ROUTE:

DISTANCE: TIME:

NOTES:

CROSS TRAINING:

TUESDAY
ROUTE:

DISTANCE: TIME:

NOTES:

CROSS TRAINING:

WEDNESDAY
ROUTE:

DISTANCE: TIME:

NOTES:

CROSS TRAINING:

THURSDAY
ROUTE:

DISTANCE: TIME:

NOTES:

CROSS TRAINING:

FRIDAY
ROUTE:

DISTANCE: TIME:

NOTES:

CROSS TRAINING:

SATURDAY

ROUTE:

DISTANCE: TIME:

NOTES:

CROSS TRAINING:

SUNDAY

ROUTE:

DISTANCE: TIME:

NOTES:

CROSS TRAINING:

NOTES

TRAINING

TEMPO RUNS

Typically, 20 minutes (or, if you go by mileage, 2 to 3 miles) is sufficient for tempo runs—if your goal is general fitness or a 5-K. Runners tackling longer distances should do longer tempo runs during their peak training weeks: 4 to 6 miles for the 10-K, 6 to 8 for the half-marathon, and 8 to 10 for 26.2. The tempo pace should feel comfortably hard, meaning that you can feel that you're working, but you're not racing. At the same time, you feel you'd be happier if you could slow down.

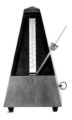

DID YOU KNOW?

A study published in 2010 in the *Journal of Strength and Conditioning Research* shows that runners who add 3 days of resistance training to their weekly program have greater upper- and lower-body strength than those who only run.

WEEKLY TOTAL

TOTAL MILEAGE TO DATE

TIP
OF THE **WEEK**

Don't be nervous about double runs. Start by doing two-a-days twice a week. Initially, the extra workout can be 20 minutes; drop the length of your main workout by 10 to 15 minutes. As you get more comfortable, bring the main workout back to its original level and extend the first run to 40 minutes. After that, you can double up on as many days as you want. Just spend at least 2 weeks at each stage before adding more miles. Allow at least 4 hours between your workouts so that you can recover fully.

"In that 2001 [post 9/11 marathon] race, more than ever, that year, that was a reminder to everybody that it is about the pursuit, the being alive, the chance to push oneself, the chance to be part of something so much greater than any individual."

—MARY WITTENBERG,
director of the New York City Marathon; president and CEO of the New York Road Runners (NYRR)

MONDAY
ROUTE:

DISTANCE: TIME:

NOTES:

CROSS TRAINING:

TUESDAY
ROUTE:

DISTANCE: TIME:

NOTES:

CROSS TRAINING:

WEDNESDAY
ROUTE:

DISTANCE: TIME:

NOTES:

CROSS TRAINING:

THURSDAY
ROUTE:

DISTANCE: TIME:

NOTES:

CROSS TRAINING:

FRIDAY
ROUTE:

DISTANCE: TIME:

NOTES:

CROSS TRAINING:

SATURDAY

ROUTE:

DISTANCE: TIME:

NOTES:

CROSS TRAINING:

SUNDAY

ROUTE:

DISTANCE: TIME:

NOTES:

CROSS TRAINING:

NOTES

WEEKLY TOTAL

TOTAL MILEAGE TO DATE

NUTRITION

DRINK UP

If you're going for a second run of the day, be sure to rehydrate, and consume at least 500 calories within 30 minutes of finishing to help speed recovery.

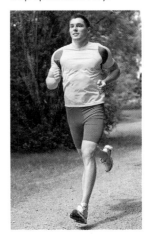

DID YOU KNOW?

The Boston Marathon is a top 50 marathons qualifier for the Boston Marathon. But to be invited back, you have to be fast enough. The acceptance of official race entrants is based on qualifying time, with the fastest qualifiers (in relation to their ages and genders) being accepted first until the race is full.

TIP
OF THE **WEEK**

Even on days you run, you should still do core work. Fortunately, it doesn't require a lot of time or equipment—just a few key moves done correctly and consistently. You can do your core workout before or after your run.

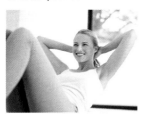

"The sense of exhilaration you feel when you're riding your pain, when after long and exacting work you've become pain's master rather than its servant, is almost indescribable."

—ALBERTO SALAZAR, New York City and Boston Marathon winner, running coach, and author of *14 Minutes: A Running Legend's Life and Death and Life*

MONDAY
ROUTE:

DISTANCE: TIME:

NOTES:

CROSS TRAINING:

TUESDAY
ROUTE:

DISTANCE: TIME:

NOTES:

CROSS TRAINING:

WEDNESDAY
ROUTE:

DISTANCE: TIME:

NOTES:

CROSS TRAINING:

THURSDAY
ROUTE:

DISTANCE: TIME:

NOTES:

CROSS TRAINING:

FRIDAY
ROUTE:

DISTANCE: TIME:

NOTES:

CROSS TRAINING:

SATURDAY

ROUTE:

DISTANCE: TIME:

NOTES:

CROSS TRAINING:

SUNDAY

ROUTE:

DISTANCE: TIME:

NOTES:

CROSS TRAINING:

NOTES

WEEKLY TOTAL

TOTAL MILEAGE TO DATE

TRAINING

DON'T IGNORE YOUR CORE

Most runners are familiar with planks and crunches, but try the "Metronome" for your oft-forgotten obliques: Lie faceup on the floor with your knees bent and raised over your hips, your ankles parallel to the ground, your feet lifted, and your arms extended outward. Rotate your legs to the left, bringing your knees as close to the floor as possible without touching it. Return to the center, then move your knees to the right. Do 10 to 12 reps on each side. Don't swing your hips or use momentum; start the movement from your core and continue to move slowly from side to side.

DID YOU KNOW?

A solid core is an important part of running performance. The muscles in the abdominals, lower back, and glutes help runners power up hills, sprint to the finish, and maintain efficient form.

TIP
OF THE **WEEK**

For every set of abdominal exercises you perform, do a set of lower-back exercises like the bird dog or cobra stretch. Focusing only on your abs can lead to poor posture and lower-back pain.

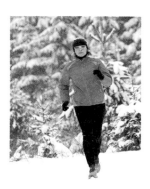

"Setting tough goals for races might mean not reaching your goals now and then. If you make an honest evaluation of why you failed, you might benefit even more than if you had achieved your goal."

—JACK DANIELS, coach and author of *Daniels' Running Formula*

MONDAY
ROUTE:

DISTANCE: TIME:

NOTES:

CROSS TRAINING:

TUESDAY
ROUTE:

DISTANCE: TIME:

NOTES:

CROSS TRAINING:

WEDNESDAY
ROUTE:

DISTANCE: TIME:

NOTES:

CROSS TRAINING:

THURSDAY
ROUTE:

DISTANCE: TIME:

NOTES:

CROSS TRAINING:

FRIDAY
ROUTE:

DISTANCE: TIME:

NOTES:

CROSS TRAINING:

SATURDAY

ROUTE:

DISTANCE: TIME:

NOTES:

CROSS TRAINING:

SUNDAY

ROUTE:

DISTANCE: TIME:

NOTES:

CROSS TRAINING:

NOTES

WEEKLY TOTAL

TOTAL MILEAGE TO DATE

TRAINING

LISTEN TO YOUR BODY

Open your inner "ears." Athletes should listen to their bodies. Pay attention to little aches and pains and even cravings. If your calf hurts after a run, figure out why. Is it time for a new pair of shoes? Do you need orthotics? And if you have a craving for salt, eat pretzels.

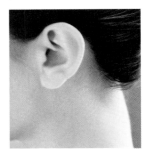

DID YOU KNOW?

Most runners don't taper properly. If you're training for a marathon, reduce your mileage by 25 percent 3 weeks before the race. Maintain that mileage 2 weeks before the race. The last week before the race, reduce your mileage again so that it's 50 percent of your normal midseason training.

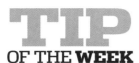

OF THE **WEEK**

If you're running a race that's a few time zones away, make sure you stay on your home time. If you're from New York and your marathon in California starts at 6 a.m. West Coast time, then wake up at 3 a.m. West Coast time, which translates to 6 a.m. in your body. Eat when you're hungry, go to bed when you're tired, and your early wake-up call will be much easier to answer.

"You have to wonder at times what you're doing out there. Over the years, I've given myself a thousand reasons to keep running, but it always comes back to where it started. It comes down to self-satisfaction and a sense of achievement."

—STEVE PREFONTAINE,
middle and distance runner;
Olympian in 5,000 m
(Munich 1972)

MONDAY
ROUTE:

DISTANCE: TIME:

NOTES:

CROSS TRAINING:

TUESDAY
ROUTE:

DISTANCE: TIME:

NOTES:

CROSS TRAINING:

WEDNESDAY
ROUTE:

DISTANCE: TIME:

NOTES:

CROSS TRAINING:

THURSDAY
ROUTE:

DISTANCE: TIME:

NOTES:

CROSS TRAINING:

FRIDAY
ROUTE:

DISTANCE: TIME:

NOTES:

CROSS TRAINING:

SATURDAY

ROUTE:

DISTANCE: TIME:

NOTES:

CROSS TRAINING:

SUNDAY

ROUTE:

DISTANCE: TIME:

NOTES:

CROSS TRAINING:

NOTES

WEEKLY TOTAL

TOTAL MILEAGE TO DATE

NUTRITION

PROTEIN PORTIONS

Athletes who don't get enough protein are at a higher risk of injury. The bad news: Vegetable-based sources, such as beans, lentils, nuts, seeds, and soy, aren't as protein-dense—$\frac{1}{2}$ cup of black beans only has about 8 grams of protein and falls short on all nine essential amino acids, the chemical building blocks of protein. (The exception to this is soy.) The good news: Lean meats and other animal products, like eggs, milk, and whey (a by-product of milk), pack a lot of protein in small portions. Four ounces of chicken breast contain about 32 grams of protein.

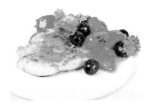

DID YOU KNOW?

A 150-pound runner doing a 4-mile training run at about a 9-minute pace burns about 480 calories.

TIP
OF THE **WEEK**

When it comes to treating your shoes right, remember: Never put them in a dryer if they're wet. Instead, remove the insoles and stuff them with newspaper. The paper will absorb the moisture and the midsoles won't be broken down by the dryer's heat.

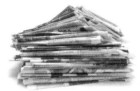

"As long as we got the best out of ourselves, we are winners. That's the definition of success. You can't say only #1 is the winner."

—MEB KEFLEZIGHI, winner of 2009 New York City marathon; 2011 US winner of Olympic marathon trials; marathon Olympic silver medalist (Athens 2004)

MONDAY
ROUTE:

DISTANCE: TIME:

NOTES:

CROSS TRAINING:

TUESDAY
ROUTE:

DISTANCE: TIME:

NOTES:

CROSS TRAINING:

WEDNESDAY
ROUTE:

DISTANCE: TIME:

NOTES:

CROSS TRAINING:

THURSDAY
ROUTE:

DISTANCE: TIME:

NOTES:

CROSS TRAINING:

FRIDAY
ROUTE:

DISTANCE: TIME:

NOTES:

CROSS TRAINING:

SATURDAY

ROUTE:

DISTANCE: TIME:

NOTES:

CROSS TRAINING:

SUNDAY

ROUTE:

DISTANCE: TIME:

NOTES:

CROSS TRAINING:

NOTES

WEEKLY TOTAL

TOTAL MILEAGE TO DATE

TRAINING

BALANCED WORKOUTS

To balance out your running workouts, try using a bike or an elliptical machine as a cross-training tool. Longer efforts add to your aerobic training volume with little stress on your body.

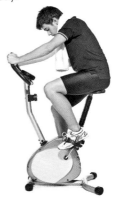

DID YOU KNOW?

Holder of the record for most marathons finished in 1 year: Larry Macon of San Antonio, Texas, who completed 105. (He averaged one marathon every 4 days in 2008.)

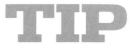

OF THE **WEEK**

If you're thinking of buying a treadmill, here are some questions you'll want to consider:

• Is it motorized (the belt is driven by an engine) or runner-driven (the runner's pace drives the belt)?

• Is the belt wide enough to accommodate your stride?

• If your machine is motorized, can the belt move as fast as you want to go?

• Does it stay in place when you hammer on it?

• Can the belt move up and down to simulate hill running?

• Do you get good traction on the belt?

• Can the computer tailor workouts to your needs?

"Triumph over adversity, that's what the marathon is all about. There's nothing in life that you can't triumph over after that."

—KATHRINE SWITZER, first woman to officially run the Boston Marathon, 1967

MONDAY
ROUTE:

DISTANCE: TIME:

NOTES:

CROSS TRAINING:

TUESDAY
ROUTE:

DISTANCE: TIME:

NOTES:

CROSS TRAINING:

WEDNESDAY
ROUTE:

DISTANCE: TIME:

NOTES:

CROSS TRAINING:

THURSDAY
ROUTE:

DISTANCE: TIME:

NOTES:

CROSS TRAINING:

FRIDAY
ROUTE:

DISTANCE: TIME:

NOTES:

CROSS TRAINING:

SATURDAY

ROUTE:

DISTANCE: TIME:

NOTES:

CROSS TRAINING:

SUNDAY

ROUTE:

DISTANCE: TIME:

NOTES:

CROSS TRAINING:

NOTES

WEEKLY TOTAL

TOTAL MILEAGE TO DATE

NUTRITION

BETTER WITH PEANUT BUTTER

One of runners' favorites, peanut butter provides a healthy dose of vitamin E. It's an ingredient in sauces, soups, casseroles, and ice cream, and it's the perfect soul mate for jelly. For a different twist on your salad tonight, whisk together peanut butter, olive oil, grated ginger, red pepper flakes, and rice vinegar to make a vinaigrette.

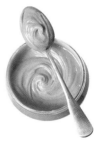

DID YOU KNOW?

According to British researchers, fit athletes who eat an energy bar containing 100 milligrams of caffeine (the amount in about 1 cup of joe) can train 27 percent longer than those who have a bar without caffeine. But stick to 100 milligrams—having more caffeine than that can cause gastrointestinal issues.

TIP
OF THE **WEEK**

Beat the post-marathon blues by walking your dog for about 30 minutes every other day. This will get you out and about while still honoring your body's need to lower your mileage for a few weeks after a marathon. If you must run, avoid hills and speedwork. This allows your damaged muscle cells to recover and helps prevent injuries. Rubbing your legs and stretching help work out the waste products that accumulate in your muscles during a marathon, so stretch daily during your post-marathon recovery period.

"The marathon can humble you."

—BILL RODGERS, 4-time winner of both Boston and New York City Marathons

MONDAY
ROUTE:

DISTANCE: TIME:

NOTES:

CROSS TRAINING:

TUESDAY
ROUTE:

DISTANCE: TIME:

NOTES:

CROSS TRAINING:

WEDNESDAY
ROUTE:

DISTANCE: TIME:

NOTES:

CROSS TRAINING:

THURSDAY
ROUTE:

DISTANCE: TIME:

NOTES:

CROSS TRAINING:

FRIDAY
ROUTE:

DISTANCE: TIME:

NOTES:

CROSS TRAINING:

SATURDAY
ROUTE:

DISTANCE: TIME:

NOTES:

CROSS TRAINING:

SUNDAY
ROUTE:

DISTANCE: TIME:

NOTES:

CROSS TRAINING:

NOTES

WEEKLY TOTAL

TOTAL MILEAGE TO DATE

TRAINING

THE TRUTH ABOUT SALT

One study found that about 30 percent of runners incorrectly believe that they need to take in extra salt while running and more than 57 percent said that they drink sports drinks because the drinks have electrolytes that prevent low blood sodium. In reality, to finish strong you need to drink only 8 to 16 ounces 1 to 2 hours before a run.

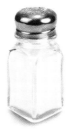

DID YOU KNOW?

Working hard to maintain your pace when running uphill is a bad strategy, according to Australian researchers. They found the effort of pushing up an incline left study subjects so tired that they lost time by running slowly after reaching the top and not going hard enough on the downhills. Focus on maintaining an even effort rather than an even pace.

TIP
OF THE **WEEK**

Keep your cell phone on you for emergencies. Even during cold weather you can overheat. If you feel light-headed, dizzy, or hot, or you experience chest pain, visual disturbances, cramping, vomiting, or headache, slow down or stop and call 911 immediately.

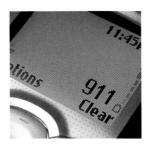

"When I first started running I was so embarrassed, I'd walk when cars passed me. I'd pretend I was looking at the flowers."

—JOAN BENOIT SAMUELSON, marathoner; 2-time Boston Marathon winner; marathon Olympic gold medalist (Los Angeles 1984)

MONDAY
ROUTE:

DISTANCE: TIME:

NOTES:

CROSS TRAINING:

TUESDAY
ROUTE:

DISTANCE: TIME:

NOTES:

CROSS TRAINING:

WEDNESDAY
ROUTE:

DISTANCE: TIME:

NOTES:

CROSS TRAINING:

THURSDAY
ROUTE:

DISTANCE: TIME:

NOTES:

CROSS TRAINING:

FRIDAY
ROUTE:

DISTANCE: TIME:

NOTES:

CROSS TRAINING:

SATURDAY
ROUTE:

DISTANCE: TIME:

NOTES:

CROSS TRAINING:

SUNDAY
ROUTE:

DISTANCE: TIME:

NOTES:

CROSS TRAINING:

NOTES

WEEKLY TOTAL

TOTAL MILEAGE TO DATE

NUTRITION

GREAT PRERUN MEAL IDEAS!

• Graham crackers and milk
• Peanut butter and whole grain waffles
• $\frac{1}{2}$ cup of Cheerios and 2 tablespoons of nuts and dried fruit

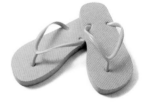

DID YOU KNOW?

Flip-flops are fine if you're wearing them for a short time (in the locker room or around the pool), but wearing them all day is unwise. Flip-flops provide no arch support, cushioning, or shock absorption, so they can lead to plantar fasciitis and shin splints.

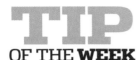

OF THE **WEEK**

Some runners suffer from GI distress and others don't simply because digestion time, hormones, stress levels, and the amount of bacteria in the stomach all affect digestion and vary between individuals. Three tips to help quell the queasiness:

1. Fiber is great, but save the bran cereals and other high-fiber foods for after your run.

2. Check the label on your sports drink or energy bar for sorbitol, mannitol, or anything ending in -ol, or fructose. These sweeteners can cause stomach upset.

3. The night before a morning run, eat dinner at least 2 hours before bed. Allow 3 hours between a big meal and your run, and try to empty your system before the race.

"The will to win is not nearly as important as the will to prepare."

—JUMA IKANGAA, marathoner from Tanzania; winner of 1986 Fukyoto Marathon and 1984 and 1986 Tokyo Marathon

MONDAY
ROUTE:

DISTANCE: TIME:

NOTES:

CROSS TRAINING:

TUESDAY
ROUTE:

DISTANCE: TIME:

NOTES:

CROSS TRAINING:

WEDNESDAY
ROUTE:

DISTANCE: TIME:

NOTES:

CROSS TRAINING:

THURSDAY
ROUTE:

DISTANCE: TIME:

NOTES:

CROSS TRAINING:

FRIDAY
ROUTE:

DISTANCE: TIME:

NOTES:

CROSS TRAINING:

SATURDAY

ROUTE:

DISTANCE: TIME:

NOTES:

CROSS TRAINING:

SUNDAY

ROUTE:

DISTANCE: TIME:

NOTES:

CROSS TRAINING:

NOTES

WEEKLY TOTAL

TOTAL MILEAGE TO DATE

TRAINING

A CURE FOR CRAMPING

If you frequently find yourself cramping up, overtraining and poor pacing could be the culprits. Researchers found that, when compared with noncrampers, runners who cramped up in South Africa's Two Oceans Marathon had run more in the 3 days prior to the race, had pre-race blood markers indicating damaged or fatigued muscles, and started the event at a more aggressive pace relative to their previous best times.

DID YOU KNOW?

Don't neglect sleep. "Athletes pay so much attention to exercise and nutrition but forget the third piece of the pie: For peak performance you need to sleep," says James Maas, PhD, a psychology professor at Cornell University. For a good night's rest, make sure to stick to a routine: Go to bed and wake up at the same time each day; keep your bedroom dark, quiet, and cool; and don't use electronic devices for 30 minutes before lights-out.

TIP OF THE WEEK

If your head hurts after a run, it could be what's called a primary exercise headache. Your risk is increased if you exercise in hot weather, exercise at high altitudes, or have a family history of migraines. Your doctor may prescribe anti-inflammatory or blood pressure medications. If, along with the headache, you're vomiting, feeling dizzy, or having double vision, make an appointment immediately.

"Blink and you miss a sprint. The 10,000 meters is lap after lap of waiting. Theatrically, the mile is just the right length—beginning, middle, end: a story unfolding."

—SEBASTIAN COE, middle distance runner, 1500 m Olympic gold medalist (Moscow 1980 and Los Angeles 1984)

MONDAY
ROUTE:

DISTANCE: TIME:

NOTES:

CROSS TRAINING:

TUESDAY
ROUTE:

DISTANCE: TIME:

NOTES:

CROSS TRAINING:

WEDNESDAY
ROUTE:

DISTANCE: TIME:

NOTES:

CROSS TRAINING:

THURSDAY
ROUTE:

DISTANCE: TIME:

NOTES:

CROSS TRAINING:

FRIDAY
ROUTE:

DISTANCE: TIME:

NOTES:

CROSS TRAINING:

SATURDAY

ROUTE:

DISTANCE: TIME:

NOTES:

CROSS TRAINING:

SUNDAY

ROUTE:

DISTANCE: TIME:

NOTES:

CROSS TRAINING:

NOTES

WEEKLY TOTAL

TOTAL MILEAGE TO DATE

NUTRITION

SQUASH SEASON!

Winter squash is a great recovery food for runners. One cup of winter squash provides 145 percent of your recommended daily intake of beta-carotene and one-third of your daily value of vitamin C. Winter squash also aids in rehydration. Most varieties are 89 percent water, and acorn squash boasts 896 milligrams of potassium per cup (nearly double that of a banana). Potassium, an electrolyte lost through sweat, helps regulate fluid levels in the body.

DID YOU KNOW?

Athletes who use instructional and motivational self-talk before and during an event perform better than those who don't, according to researchers in Greece. Try it: Review your race strategy; tell yourself how you plan to achieve your goal. Repeat a mantra (such as "Start out slow" or "I am tough") as you run.

TRAINING

Having trouble getting your runs in? Do them first thing in the morning, before the day begins. With no meetings, meals to make, or errands to run, early morning is a great time to ensure that you get your run done.

The night before, set the coffeemaker to brew before you wake. Lay your clothes out by the door. Arrange an early morning running date. Turn off the computer 30 minutes before bed. In the morning, get dressed in a brightly lit room; when the light hits your eyes, it signals your pineal gland to stop producing melatonin, a hormone that makes you feel sleepy.

"My fiercest competition was always myself. If I could reach into the depths of my capabilities and perform to the greatest extent I was capable of on a given day, based on proper preparation, that's all I could ask of myself."

—**BILLY MILLS,** Olympic 10,000 m bronze medalist (Tokyo 1964) and Native American humanitarian

MONDAY
ROUTE:

DISTANCE: TIME:

NOTES:

CROSS TRAINING:

TUESDAY
ROUTE:

DISTANCE: TIME:

NOTES:

CROSS TRAINING:

WEDNESDAY
ROUTE:

DISTANCE: TIME:

NOTES:

CROSS TRAINING:

THURSDAY
ROUTE:

DISTANCE: TIME:

NOTES:

CROSS TRAINING:

FRIDAY
ROUTE:

DISTANCE: TIME:

NOTES:

CROSS TRAINING:

SATURDAY

ROUTE:

DISTANCE: TIME:

NOTES:

CROSS TRAINING:

SUNDAY

ROUTE:

DISTANCE: TIME:

NOTES:

CROSS TRAINING:

NOTES

WEEKLY TOTAL

TOTAL MILEAGE TO DATE

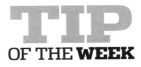

OF THE **WEEK**

You want to run in new shoes for 2 weeks and ideally have at least one long run in them before any race.

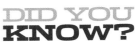

KNOW?

British researchers found that triathletes who set high goals finished an Olympic-distance race faster than those who didn't set ambitious targets. Additionally, athletes who were motivated to perform better than others clocked faster times than competitors whose aim was just to avoid doing worse than others.

TIP
OF THE **WEEK**

When you're running in the dark, don't leave home without a headlamp or handheld light. The whitish beam is a color the eye sees clearly at night. And with your motion causing the light to move—the headlamp a little, the handheld a lot—a driver should recognize you as a runner.

"There is a great advantage in training under unfavorable conditions. It is better to train under bad conditions, for the difference is then a tremendous relief in a race."

—EMIL ZÁTOPEK, Czech distance and marathon runner, 3-time Olympic gold medalist (Helsinki 1952)

MONDAY
ROUTE:

DISTANCE: TIME:

NOTES:

CROSS TRAINING:

TUESDAY
ROUTE:

DISTANCE: TIME:

NOTES:

CROSS TRAINING:

WEDNESDAY
ROUTE:

DISTANCE: TIME:

NOTES:

CROSS TRAINING:

THURSDAY
ROUTE:

DISTANCE: TIME:

NOTES:

CROSS TRAINING:

FRIDAY
ROUTE:

DISTANCE: TIME:

NOTES:

CROSS TRAINING:

SATURDAY

ROUTE:

DISTANCE: TIME:

NOTES:

CROSS TRAINING:

SUNDAY

ROUTE:

DISTANCE: TIME:

NOTES:

CROSS TRAINING:

NOTES

WEEKLY TOTAL

TOTAL MILEAGE TO DATE

NUTRITION

EATING SMART FOR RACE DAY

Many runners make the mistake of topping off their glycogen stores by feasting on carbs in the form of a spaghetti dinner the night before a race. But flooding your system with more carbs than it can process may lead to digestive problems that will have you running to the toilet every mile. Consume moderate quantities of carbs for several days prior to your race, and spread your consumption out throughout each day. Have oatmeal for breakfast, potatoes at lunch, and a small pasta dinner.

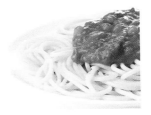

DID YOU KNOW?

After age 30, inactive adults will lose 3 to 5 percent of their muscle mass per decade. But as long you stimulate muscles, that loss is minimized.

TIP
OF THE **WEEK**

Don't hang on to your old running shoes (those past 300 to 500 miles) for walking if they're worn unevenly. To determine whether they are, set your old running shoes on a table. If they tilt to one side or wobble easily from side to side when you nudge them, then they've worn unevenly and should be recycled and replaced.

"At the two-thirds mark, I think of those who are still with me. Who might make a break? Should I? Then I give it all I've got."

—IBRAHIM HUSSEIN, the first African to win the Boston Marathon ('88, '91, '92)

MONDAY
ROUTE:

DISTANCE: TIME:

NOTES:

CROSS TRAINING:

TUESDAY
ROUTE:

DISTANCE: TIME:

NOTES:

CROSS TRAINING:

WEDNESDAY
ROUTE:

DISTANCE: TIME:

NOTES:

CROSS TRAINING:

THURSDAY
ROUTE:

DISTANCE: TIME:

NOTES:

CROSS TRAINING:

FRIDAY
ROUTE:

DISTANCE: TIME:

NOTES:

CROSS TRAINING:

SATURDAY

ROUTE:

DISTANCE: TIME:

NOTES:

CROSS TRAINING:

SUNDAY

ROUTE:

DISTANCE: TIME:

NOTES:

CROSS TRAINING:

NOTES

WEEKLY TOTAL

TOTAL MILEAGE TO DATE

TRAINING

TAKE TO THE HILLS

Rethink hills by taking them piecemeal. Run 10 easy minutes to the base of a small hill with a very gradual downhill side. Walk to the top, turn around, and count 40 to 50 steps back down. Start your first hill acceleration there: Jog for 10 to 20 steps, then pick up the pace as you reach the top of the hill. Increase your turnover and let gravity pull you down the other side. Walk or jog back to the starting point and repeat. Start with two hills and slowly work up to six.

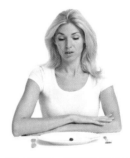

DID YOU KNOW?

Don't try to starve yourself today to make up for overeating yesterday. Get back on track with a smart breakfast—300 to 400 calories of high-quality carbohydrates, low-fat dairy, and fruit.

TIP
OF THE **WEEK**

The key to evening racing is to eat enough without overdoing it, so you don't feel full while running. Eat a hearty breakfast and a lighter lunch that's low in fat and fiber to avoid digestive trouble. Have a 300-calorie snack at 3 or 4 p.m., giving your body time to process the food before the race. Choose easily digested carbs, such as a sports drink, raisins, and a few whole grain crackers.

"Plan for what's in your capabilities. You can talk a big game and you can stick your chest out and act like you're a tough guy, but you're going to be dropped and you're going to have a miserable experience if you go out too hard."

—ALAN CULPEPPER,
distance and marathon runner,
2-time Olympian

MONDAY
ROUTE:

DISTANCE:　　　　　　　　　　　　TIME:

NOTES:

CROSS TRAINING:

TUESDAY
ROUTE:

DISTANCE:　　　　　　　　　　　　TIME:

NOTES:

CROSS TRAINING:

WEDNESDAY
ROUTE:

DISTANCE:　　　　　　　　　　　　TIME:

NOTES:

CROSS TRAINING:

THURSDAY
ROUTE:

DISTANCE:　　　　　　　　　　　　TIME:

NOTES:

CROSS TRAINING:

FRIDAY
ROUTE:

DISTANCE:　　　　　　　　　　　　TIME:

NOTES:

CROSS TRAINING:

SATURDAY

ROUTE:

DISTANCE: TIME:

NOTES:

CROSS TRAINING:

SUNDAY

ROUTE:

DISTANCE: TIME:

NOTES:

CROSS TRAINING:

NOTES

WEEKLY TOTAL

TOTAL MILEAGE TO DATE

NUTRITION

BE AN EARLY BIRD

If you get too nervous to eat before a race, wake up a few hours before the start so you can eat breakfast slowly, letting each bite settle before taking another. If you can't stomach solid foods, drink a smoothie made with bananas, fruit juice, and milk. These ingredients are easy on most stomachs, provide energy, and won't leave you feeling overly full.

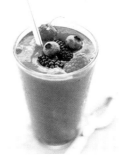

DID YOU KNOW?

Dehydration can result in slower times, while overdrinking can lead to hyponatremia, a dangerous condition where sodium levels are diluted. Ideally, you should drink 8 to 16 ounces of fluid 2 hours prior to a race. If your urine is pale yellow, you're drinking enough.

TIP OF THE **WEEK**

If you still have a few pounds you just can't seem to lose, you don't necessarily have to run more. Adding miles may increase your risk for injury. Instead, add strength training to your exercise routine. If you increase your lean muscle mass, you'll increase your body's ability to use oxygen and burn more calories.

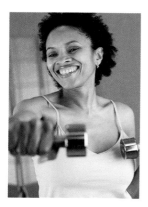

"I have fought the good fight, I have finished the race, I have kept the faith."

—2 TIMOTHY 4:7
(Paul of Tarsus)

MONDAY
ROUTE:

DISTANCE: TIME:

NOTES:

CROSS TRAINING:

TUESDAY
ROUTE:

DISTANCE: TIME:

NOTES:

CROSS TRAINING:

WEDNESDAY
ROUTE:

DISTANCE: TIME:

NOTES:

CROSS TRAINING:

THURSDAY
ROUTE:

DISTANCE: TIME:

NOTES:

CROSS TRAINING:

FRIDAY
ROUTE:

DISTANCE: TIME:

NOTES:

CROSS TRAINING:

SATURDAY

ROUTE:

DISTANCE: TIME:

NOTES:

CROSS TRAINING:

SUNDAY

ROUTE:

DISTANCE: TIME:

NOTES:

CROSS TRAINING:

NOTES

WEEKLY TOTAL

TOTAL MILEAGE TO DATE

TRAINING

STAVE OFF SORENESS

If weight training makes you sore the next day, you're probably lifting too much. Focus on building muscular endurance—rather than brute strength—by doing more repetitions with less weight. Complete two or three sets of at least 20 reps of each exercise. Work your way up to 30 repetitions *before* increasing the weight. End each of your sessions when you feel worked, but not exhausted.

DID YOU KNOW?

Studies have shown that runners are at increased risk for malignant melanomas. Avoid running from 10 a.m. to 4 p.m.; that's when the most potent ultraviolet rays shine. The impact of the sun can be amplified if you're running in an area surrounded by snow. Wear sunglasses and a hat to stay covered. Guys should keep their shirts on while running; women should avoid running just in jogbras. Look for running clothing that offers UV protection, or wear darker colors, which block more UV rays than light colors. Use sunscreen with an SPF of 30+ and labeled "broad spectrum."

NOW WHAT?
YOUR YEAR IN REVIEW

Congratulations. You've reached the end of your running year. Now it's time for a quick review. Did you reach your goals? Ah, goals. So easy to set; so tough to achieve.

This isn't the place for a lecture on goal setting. You need only remember three things: be specific, be realistic, and be wide-ranging. Don't focus exclusively on your training mileage or race times. Take a broader approach—one that considers health and motivation. By using this training journal as your number-one friend, motivator, and coach—especially now, at the end of the year—you can reach your goals, any and all.

1. LOOK BACK TO YOUR BEST RACE DURING THE YEAR. In running, there's no such thing as a "lucky" day. You did something right—probably weeks and months of good choices and training techniques. List them and save the list.

2. FIND THE 4-WEEK PERIOD WHEN YOU RAN THE MOST MILES. Try to figure out why this period worked so well for you. Why were other weeks less successful? In the coming year, copy the positive; eliminate the negative.

3. TRACE THE COURSE OF ANY INJURIES YOU HAD DURING THE YEAR. Which came from accidents? Potholes in the road? Find a detour. Bad shoes? Don't buy them again.

4. TRY TO DETERMINE WHAT HELPS YOU RUN THE BEST. Were you up at the crack of dawn? Was it the challenge of the race? Did you find a running buddy? Help with a charity event? You'll see the pattern of what motivated you to lace up your shoes.

5. MAKE A SEASONAL PLAN FOR THE COMING YEAR. You can't know what's going to happen to you in the next 12 months. But you'll have a better chance of achieving your running and fitness goals if you choose the basic path you hope to follow.

6. ADD AT LEAST ONE NEW EXERCISE TO YOUR WORKOUT REPERTOIRE. Start strength training. Buy a mountain bike. Learn to swim. Consider snowshoeing. Every new workout makes your fitness foundation stronger.

7. PICK SEVERAL NEW RACES TO ENTER IN THE COMING YEAR. Try a trail race or a mountain race. Get a few friends together for a road relay. Or simply enter some races or race distances you've never tackled before.

8. BUY ANOTHER TRAINING DIARY. Scientific studies have proven the power of putting things down in writing. For a runner, that means a training diary.

SHOES

The beauty of running as a sport is that you don't need a lot of gear to get started or to enjoy it (especially if you're a veteran). But don't pinch pennies when you're shopping for running shoes. Running in shoes that don't fit right or that have too many miles on them will lead to injuries. If the shoe fits *you* well—buy it. As a rule, we recommend recyling your shoes once they've got 300–500 miles on them. Some shoes may last longer. But if you've abused them with trail debris, hot roads, or lots of puddles, get rid of them sooner. Better yet, get two pairs of the same kind of running shoe and use them on alternate runs. It may take a few false starts to find the shoes that are right for you. Use the next few pages to record information on the shoes you ran in this year. It will help you dial in to the model that's best for you. (It's likely you'll need to buy two or three pairs of running shoes per year.)

Shoe name (Nike Air Max, Asics Gel-Kayano, etc.): _____

_____

Date purchased: _____ Price: _____

Size: _____

Where you bought it: _____

Foot size (measured—yes? no?): _____

Date you started using this shoe: _____

Date you retired shoe from active duty: _____

Miles of use: _____

Impressions: _____

Shoe name (Nike Air Max, Asics Gel-Kayano, etc.): _____

_____

Date purchased: _____ Price: _____

Size: _____

Where you bought it: _____

Foot size (measured—yes? no?): _____

Date you started using this shoe: _____

Date you retired shoe from active duty: _____

Miles of use: _____

Impressions: _____

Shoe name (Nike Air Max, Asics Gel-Kayano, etc.): _____

_____

Date purchased: _____ Price: _____

Size: _____

Where you bought it: _____

Foot size (measured—yes? no?): _____

Date you started using this shoe: _____

Date you retired shoe from active duty: _____

Miles of use: _____

Impressions: _____

Shoeless?

Maybe this was the year you decided to be a minimalist: just running shorts and the open road. Any time you can put your feet in control of their movement, it's usually a good thing. Whether you decide on the barest of footwear or foot gloves, your experience will be unlike anything you've ever known before. Write it down. Both shod and minimalist running have their drawbacks. Keep track of what you thought were the positive and negative qualities of each.

Minimal shoe name (Merrell Barefoot, Saucony Kinvara, etc.): _____

_____

Date purchased: _____ Price: _____

Size: _____

Where you bought it: _____

Foot size (measured—yes? no?): _____

Date you started using this shoe: _____

Date you retired shoe from active duty: _____

Miles of use: _____

Impressions: _____

RAVE RUNS
THE PATHS YOU RAN

What makes a run memorable? The answers are as different as runners themselves. Maybe it's the trail, the road, the scenery, or the way the city looks
throughout the seasons. Maybe it's your companion and the conversation you had.
Maybe you achieved a PR on a regular course or ran more distance than ever before.
Maybe it's a combination of all of the above. Then again, you may have had a run
that was pure drudgery. You sprained an ankle. You had a fight with your running
buddy (and she's still not talking to you). But running is about taking the good with
the bad and what you take away from both. Record your rave and rotten runs here.

Date: _____ Route: _____

Miles: _____ Time: _____

Companions? _____

Chat? _____

Weather: _____

Why was this run so great or horrible? _____

Date: _____ Route: _____

Miles: _____ Time: _____

Companions? _____

Chat? _____

Weather: _____

Why was this run so great or horrible? _____

Date: _____ Route: _____

Miles: _____ Time: _____

Companions? _____

Chat? _____

Weather: _____

Why was this run so great or horrible? _____

Date: _____ Route: _____

Miles: _____ Time: _____

Companions? _____

Chat? _____

Weather: _____

Why was this run so great or horrible? _____

Date: _____ Route: _____

Miles: _____ Time: _____

Companions? _____

Chat? _____

Weather: _____

Why was this run so great or horrible? _____

Date: _____ Route: _____

Miles: _____ Time: _____

Companions? _____

Chat? _____

Weather: _____

Why was this run so great or horrible? _____

Date: _____ Route: _____

Miles: _____ Time: _____

Companions? _____

Chat? _____

Weather: _____

Why was this run so great or horrible? _____

Date: _____ Route: _____

Miles: _____ Time: _____

Companions? _____

Chat? _____

Weather: _____

Why was this run so great or horrible? _____

Date: _____ Route: _____

Miles: _____ Time: _____

Companions? _____

Chat? _____

Weather: _____

Why was this run so great or horrible? _____

Date: _____ Route: _____

Miles: _____ Time: _____

Companions? _____

Chat? _____

Weather: _____

Why was this run so great or horrible? _____

Date: _____ Route: _____

Miles: _____ Time: _____

Companions? _____

Chat? _____

Weather: _____

Why was this run so great or horrible? _____

Date: _____ Route: _____

Miles: _____ Time: _____

Companions? _____

Chat? _____

Weather: _____

Why was this run so great or horrible? _____

Date: _____ Route: _____

Miles: _____ Time: _____

Companions? _____

Chat? _____

Weather: _____

Why was this run so great or horrible? _____

Date: _____ Route: _____

Miles: _____ Time: _____

Companions? _____

Chat? _____

Weather: _____

Why was this run so great or horrible? _____

Date: _____   Route: _____

Miles: _____   Time: _____

Companions? _____

Chat? _____

Weather: _____

Why was this run so great or horrible? _____

Date: _____   Route: _____

Miles: _____   Time: _____

Companions? _____

Chat? _____

Weather: _____

Why was this run so great or horrible? _____

Date: _____   Route: _____

Miles: _____   Time: _____

Companions? _____

Chat? _____

Weather: _____

Why was this run so great or horrible? _____

Date: _____ Route: _____

Miles: _____ Time: _____

Companions? _____

Chat? _____

Weather: _____

Why was this run so great or horrible? _____

Date: _____ Route: _____

Miles: _____ Time: _____

Companions? _____

Chat? _____

Weather: _____

Why was this run so great or horrible? _____

Date: _____ Route: _____

Miles: _____ Time: _____

Companions? _____

Chat? _____

Weather: _____

Why was this run so great or horrible? _____

Date: _____   Route: _____

Miles: _____   Time: _____

Companions? _____

Chat? _____

Weather: _____

Why was this run so great or horrible? _____

Date: _____   Route: _____

Miles: _____   Time: _____

Companions? _____

Chat? _____

Weather: _____

Why was this run so great or horrible? _____

Date: _____   Route: _____

Miles: _____   Time: _____

Companions? _____

Chat? _____

Weather: _____

Why was this run so great or horrible? _____

Date: _____ Route: _____

Miles: _____ Time: _____

Companions? _____

Chat? _____

Weather: _____

Why was this run so great or horrible? _____

Date: _____ Route: _____

Miles: _____ Time: _____

Companions? _____

Chat? _____

Weather: _____

Why was this run so great or horrible? _____

Date: _____ Route: _____

Miles: _____ Time: _____

Companions? _____

Chat? _____

Weather: _____

Why was this run so great or horrible? _____

Date: _____   Route: _____

Miles: _____   Time: _____

Companions? _____

Chat? _____

Weather: _____

Why was this run so great or horrible? _____

Date: _____   Route: _____

Miles: _____   Time: _____

Companions? _____

Chat? _____

Weather: _____

Why was this run so great or horrible? _____

Date: _____   Route: _____

Miles: _____   Time: _____

Companions? _____

Chat? _____

Weather: _____

Why was this run so great or horrible? _____

RACE PERFORMANCE

Whether you're a veteran or you're new to running, if you train safe, racing should be a part of your running experience. Participating in a race is an excellent running goal. You get to put yourself and your fitness to the test, you come together with a community of like-minded people, and your training gains focus. You can run to meet a goal, or run for a charity or a cause. And then there are the T-shirts. Record your race performances on the next few pages.

Race name: _____ Town: _____

Distance: _____

Course description: _____

Your time: _____

Your place overall: _____

Age group place: _____

Describe the whole experience: _____

Race name: _____ Town: _____

Distance: _____

Course description: _____

Your time: _____

Your place overall: _____

Age group place: _____

Describe the whole experience: _____

Race name: _____   Town: _____

Distance: _____

Course description: _____

Your time: _____

Your place overall: _____

Age group place: _____

Describe the whole experience: _____

Race name: _____   Town: _____

Distance: _____

Course description: _____

Your time: _____

Your place overall: _____

Age group place: _____

Describe the whole experience: _____

Race name: _____ Town: _____

Distance: _____

Course description: _____

Your time: _____

Your place overall: _____

Age group place: _____

Describe the whole experience: _____

Race name: _____ Town: _____

Distance: _____

Course description: _____

Your time: _____

Your place overall: _____

Age group place: _____

Describe the whole experience: _____

Race name: _____   Town: _____

Distance: _____

Course description: _____

Your time: _____

Your place overall: _____

Age group place: _____

Describe the whole experience: _____

Race name: _____   Town: _____

Distance: _____

Course description: _____

Your time: _____

Your place overall: _____

Age group place: _____

Describe the whole experience: _____

Race name: _____ Town: _____

Distance: _____

Course description: _____

Your time: _____

Your place overall: _____

Age group place: _____

Describe the whole experience: _____

Race name: _____ Town: _____

Distance: _____

Course description: _____

Your time: _____

Your place overall: _____

Age group place: _____

Describe the whole experience: _____

Race name: _____ Town: _____

Distance: _____

Course description: _____

Your time: _____

Your place overall: _____

Age group place: _____

Describe the whole experience: _____

Race name: _____ Town: _____

Distance: _____

Course description: _____

Your time: _____

Your place overall: _____

Age group place: _____

Describe the whole experience: _____

Race name: _____ Town: _____

Distance: _____

Course description: _____

Your time: _____

Your place overall: _____

Age group place: _____

Describe the whole experience: _____

Race name: _____ Town: _____

Distance: _____

Course description: _____

Your time: _____

Your place overall: _____

Age group place: _____

Describe the whole experience: _____

Race name: _____ Town: _____

Distance: _____

Course description: _____

Your time: _____

Your place overall: _____

Age group place: _____

Describe the whole experience: _____

Race name: _____ Town: _____

Distance: _____

Course description: _____

Your time: _____

Your place overall: _____

Age group place: _____

Describe the whole experience: _____

Race name: _____ Town: _____

Distance: _____

Course description: _____

Your time: _____

Your place overall: _____

Age group place: _____

Describe the whole experience: _____

Race name: _____ Town: _____

Distance: _____

Course description: _____

Your time: _____

Your place overall: _____

Age group place: _____

Describe the whole experience: _____

Race name: _____   Town: _____

Distance: _____

Course description: _____

Your time: _____

Your place overall: _____

Age group place: _____

Describe the whole experience: _____

Race name: _____   Town: _____

Distance: _____

Course description: _____

Your time: _____

Your place overall: _____

Age group place: _____

Describe the whole experience: _____

TRAINING PLANS

In this edition of the *Runner's World Training Journal,* we've gathered some of the best training plans for the most popular race distances. No matter what your goals are—finishing a marathon, losing weight, running faster or longer—you can find more great resources in the *Runner's World* books cited at the end of this journal or online at runnersworld.com.

TRAINING PROGRAM: YOUR BEST 5-K EVER

The 5-K is a great distance for every level of runner. It's fail-safe short for fidgety first-timers. There's one nearly every weekend for personal record–chasing intermediates. And it's the ideal fast time trial, tough tempo run, or 10-K-to-marathon tune-up for veteran competitors.

We've included a 5-week schedule for each of the three groups (beginner, intermediate, and advanced). You'll also see the "Four 5-K Training Universals" on page 131. Check these out before getting to your schedule, as these principles apply to everyone.

Have a look at the three training levels below to determine which describes you best, and therefore which schedule you should follow.

BEGINNER: You're running recreationally two or three times a week for a total of 6 to 8-plus miles, and you've done a few fun-run shorties. But now you want to enter a real race—and finish. Join the order of road racers. Score that first race T-shirt. Earn some bragging rights at the office.

INTERMEDIATE: You've been running consistently for at least a year and have run in a few races, but mainly for the experience. You've dabbled in some modest interval training. Now you want to think seriously about your finishing time and how to lower it: to race, not just participate.

ADVANCED: You have at least several years of serious running behind you, follow a year-round schedule, have run in many races at various distances, have done regular interval training, want to discover your personal performance ceiling, and are willing to push hard in training.

Four 5-K Training Universals

1. REST
No running at all. Walk, bike, or swim, if you want to—just not very hard. Don't think of rest days as "nothing" days, but rather as a different kind of training that allows your body to recover while it absorbs and consolidates the strength gains your hard runs produce.

2. EASY RUNS
These should be totally comfortable. You're breathing hard enough to know that you're running, but still able to hold up your end of an on-the-run chat. If you can't, it's too hard. On the other hand, if you can sing every verse of "Old MacDonald Had a Farm" en route, it's too easy.

3. LONG RUNS
Long runs are a key training tool. Their purpose is to build endurance, specifically the ability to run for longer and longer periods of time without crapping out.

4. SPEED (INTERVALS, TEMPO)
Speed runs are shorter than race distance repetitions at or below your goal race pace. These can be hard to very hard to nearly all-out. Speed workouts produce leg speed, elevated lactic threshold, stamina, biomechanical efficiency, and the ability to tolerate the discomfort that's essential to racing fitness.

Beginner

At this stage, you just run. A little more this week than the week before, a tad more during the week that follows. No interval training, no flirting with injuries, no serious discomfort. Just run.

"For runners without a competitive past, the first training goal is to raise mileage by adding easy volume," says former US Olympian and Internet coach Jon Sinclair (anaerobic.net). "First of all, it develops increased aerobic conditioning, which by itself yields faster times. Second, it produces the physical strength on which later, harder training can be built."

What about speed training at this level? "Not a good idea," says Sinclair. "Adding any intensity in the form of fartleks or hills to a person's program can be dangerous and counterproductive. At this stage in a runner's development, the first rule should be 'Do no harm.' If they just run more, they will, in a few months, run faster."

REMEMBER: Every run in this 5-week schedule should be a steady run, done at an effort that has you breathing "comfortably hard," but way, way short of squinty-eyed wheezing. Enjoy each run, feel yourself getting stronger and leaner, and be proud of what you're doing.

Beginner 5-K Training Plan

WEEK	MON	TUES	WED	THURS	FRI	SAT	SUN
1	Rest	1.5 miles easy	Rest	1.5 miles easy	Rest	2 miles easy	Rest
2	Rest	2 miles easy	Rest	2 miles easy	Rest	2.5 miles easy	Rest
3	Rest	2 miles easy	Rest	2.5 miles easy	Rest	3 miles easy	Rest
4	Rest	2.5 miles easy	Rest	2.5 miles easy	Rest	3 miles easy	Rest
5	Rest	2.5 miles easy	Rest	2 miles easy	Rest	Rest	Race Day

Race Day Rules

"For a beginner, expending energy in a race can be scary and looked upon as a big barrier," says Portland, Oregon–based coach Bob Williams. "But if you've run at least that long in training many times, and run negative splits—first half slower than the second—in the race, you'll enjoy the experience and finish feeling good."

Have an energy bar and some fluids for breakfast, then arrive early so you can pick up your race number and avoid the drain of long lines. Do a little warmup by walking and jogging, sip some water, stretch a bit, and generally hang out and stay stress-free until the start. Remind yourself that your goal is to finish, to run the whole way, and to finish feeling tired—but not trashed.

Racing Flats

Will they make you faster? Yes. Studies have shown that if the load on your feet is lightened by 200 grams (about 6 ounces, the weight difference between training shoes and racing flats), you'll take 1 to 2 percent less time to cover a given distance—so, for a 24-minute 5-K, you can shave 12 to 20 seconds off your time by wearing racing flats. But, it's never a good idea to wear something different in your race for the first time. Wear those flats once a week for 2 to 3 weeks before racing in them.

Intermediate

To segue from finisher to racer, you'll need to add more weekly miles, yes, but more important, you'll need to add intensity in the form of timed intervals both at (pace intervals) and below (speed intervals) your 5-K goal pace. You may also want to add a hill-training session every other week.

"Running hills once a week—a 5 to 6 grade is optimal—at a fairly hard effort for up to 3 minutes at a time is an ideal way to get stronger," says Sinclair. How come? Because hill training greatly improves leg and gluteal strength while increasing aerobic capacity and stride length, along with ankle flexion that enables you to "pop" off the ground more quickly.

How hard is "fairly hard"? A classic study from years ago found that running up even a slight hill at a steady pace raises your heart rate up to 26 beats higher than the same effort on flat ground. So 5-K effort (not pace) is what to shoot for.

Again, regarding intensity as opposed to mileage, a recent study in the online journal *Peak Performance* found that you'll run your best races, from 5-K up, not when you've run the most miles, but when you hit a reasonable mileage level and then crank up your intensity.

Intermediate 5-K Training Plan

WEEK	M	T	W	T	F	S	S
1	3 miles plus 5 × strides	Rest	1 mile easy 2 miles with PI 1 mile easy	Rest	3 miles plus 5 × strides	3 to 4 miles; 15-min core workout	Rest
2	3 miles plus 7 × strides	Rest	1 mile easy 2 miles with PI 1 mile easy	Rest	3 miles plus 5 × strides	5 to 6 miles; 15-min core workout	Rest
3	3 miles plus 9 × strides	Rest	1 mile easy 3 miles with PI 1 mile easy	Rest	3 miles plus 6 × strides	6 miles; 15-min core workout	Rest
4	3 miles plus 10 × strides	Rest	1 mile easy 3 miles with PI 1 mile easy	Rest	3 miles plus 5 × strides	6 miles; 15-min core workout	Rest
5	3 miles plus 10 × strides	Rest	3 miles easy with 15-min core workout	Rest	2 miles easy	2 miles plus 3 × strides	1 mile easy 4 × strides 5-K Race 1 mile easy

Stuff You Need to Know

PACE INTERVALS (PI) If your 5-K goal is 10:00 pace (31:02 finishing time), run pace intervals at 1:15 (for 200 meters), 2:30 (400 m), 5:00 (800 m). For 9:00 goal pace (27:56), it's 1:07 (200 m), 2:15 (400 m), 4:30 (800 m). For 8:00 goal pace (24:50), it's 1:00 (200 m), 2:00 (400 m), 4:00 (800 m). For 7:00 goal pace (21:44), it's 0:53 (200 m), 1:45 (400 m), 3:30 (800 m).

RECOVERY TIME For pace intervals, slowly jog half the distance of the repetition (200 m jog after 400 m repetitions).

HILLS AND EASY RUNS For 9:00 pace, use the lower number; 7:00 folks move toward the higher.

INTERVAL AND HILL DAYS Jog 1 mile, then run 4 × 100 m strides to get primed before the workout. Jog 1 mile to cool down after, then stretch.

STRIDE (S) Gradually pick up speed to 90 percent effort, hold that for 60 yards, then decelerate. Do four to six repetitions of 100 m after Wednesday and/or Saturday runs.

Race Day Rules

"It's all about negative splits," says Williams. "Always." Which means you run the first half of the race slower than the second half. Tough to do when you're pumped up, but you must. Hold back in the first mile, Williams advises, then "seek out other runners to pass in the second mile, but don't push beyond a comfortably hard effort." Increase gradually to discomfort during the last mile, and over the final 400 meters, try to pick it up.

Advanced

Two words define the training goal at this stage of your running life: "race feel." To reach your 5-K ceiling, you must replicate in training how it feels to run that far, that fast. That means timed intervals both at (pace) and faster than (speed) your 5-K goal pace—but with short recoveries. Uncomfortably short because in a race, of course, there is no recovery. So the more intimate you become with the sensations of the race itself on a twice-weekly basis, the more you'll be able to handle the 5-K's physical and mental combination punches on race day.

You have legendary British coach Frank Horwill to thank for this. Horwill found that when athletes were stuck at a certain 5-K time—sometimes for years—and could not break through, they were almost always running lots of repetitions significantly faster than 5-K race pace (sometimes as fast as 56 seconds) with 400-meter jogs. When Horwill pointed out that they would not get 400-meter recovery periods in a race, the usual reply was "But I'm running so much faster than race pace." Sorry, Horwill said, it doesn't work that way.

Invariably, when he had his runners do the repeats slightly faster than their projected 5-K pace, with recovery jogs as short as 50 meters (about 20 seconds), their times dropped. "They needed to get the feel of what it was like to run a tough 5-K race," Horwill explained. "The recovery time after repetitions at 5-K pace is a crucial factor." Figure to jog a quarter to a half of the distance of the repetition.

Stuff You Need to Know

PACE INTERVALS For 8:00 pace (24:50 finishing time), run 1:00 (for 200 meters), 1:30 (300 m), 2:00 (400 m), 4:00 (800 m), 6:00 (1200 m). For 6:00 pace (18:38), run 0:45 (200 m), 1:07 (300 m), 1:30 (400 m), 3:00 (800 m), 4:30 (1200 m).

SPEED INTERVALS For 8:00 pace, run 0:56 (200 m), 1:19 (300 m), 1:52 (400 m), 3:44 (800 m), 5:38 (1200 m). For 6:00 pace, run 0:41 (200 m), 1:01 (300 m), 1:22 (400 m), 2:44 (800 m), 4:08 (1200 m).

STRIDES (S): Gradually pick up speed to about 90 percent effort; hold that for 60 yards, then decelerate. Walk to full recovery before you start the next one. Nothing big, nothing really stressful—just enough to let your body go, "Ah, so this is what it feels like to go fast."

RECOVERY TIME For pace intervals, jog a quarter the distance of the repetition (100 m jog after 400 m repetitions). For speed intervals, jog half the distance.

INTERVAL AND HILL DAYS Jog 2 miles to warm up, then do 4 × 100 m strides to get primed for the workout. Jog 2 miles to cool down, then stretch.

Advanced 5-K Training Plan

WEEK	M	T	W	T	F	S	S
1	Day Off-Rest	Run 2 × 1200 meters & 2 × 800 meters at RACE-PACE. Run 4 × 100 meters strides.*	Run 4 to 6 miles EASY (at a pace easy enough to hold a conversation)	Run 2 × 800 meters, 2 × 400 meters, and 4 × 200 meters at speed pace (about 30 seconds faster per mile than your race pace)	Day Off-Rest	Run 4 to 6 miles EASY	Run 7 to 9 miles EASY
2	Day Off-Rest	Run 10 × 300 meters intervals at RACE PACE. Run 4 × 100 meters strides.*	Run 4 to 6 miles EASY	Run 1 × 800 meters, 2 × 400 meters, & 4 × 200 meters at RACE PACE	Day Off-Rest	Run 4 to 6 miles EASY	Run 7 to 9 miles EASY
3	Day Off-Rest	Run 2 × 1200 meters intervals, 2 × 800 meters intervals at RACE-PACE. Run 4 × 400 meters strides.*	Run 4 to 6 miles EASY	Run 2 × 800 meters intervals, 4 × 400 meters intervals, & 4 × 200 meters intervals at SPEED PACE	Day Off-Rest	Run 4 to 6 miles EASY	Run 8 to 10 miles EASY
4	Day Off-Rest	Run 3 × 800 meter intervals at SPEED PACE. Run 4 × 100 meters strides.*	Run 4 to 6 miles EASY	Run 3 × 800 meters, 3 × 400 meters, & 3 × 200 meters at SPEED PACE. Run 2 × 100 meters strides	Day Off-Rest	Run 4 to 6 miles EASY	Run 8 to 10 miles EASY
5	Day Off-Rest	Run 2 × 1200 meters, 2 × 800 meters, 2 × 400 meters, & 2 × 200 meters at RACE PACE*	Run 4 to 6 miles EASY	Run 4 × 400 meters, 4 × 300 meters, & 4 × 200 meters at SPEED PACE. Run 4 × 100 meters strides.	Day Off-Rest	Run 4 to 6 miles EASY	Run 8 to 10 miles EASY
6	Day Off-Rest	Run 2 × 400 metrs, 2 × 300 meters, & 2 × 200 meters at SPEED PACE. Run 6 × 100 meters strides.	Run 3 miles EASY	Run 4 × 200 meters at speed pace and 4 × 100 meters strides	Day Off-Rest	Run 2 miles EASY	Run: 5-K Race

*May replace this workout with hill training.

TRAINING PROGRAM: YOUR ULTIMATE 10-K PLAN

Training for a 10-K provides all-around fitness. It includes ample amounts of the three core components of distance running—strength, stamina, and speed. You can use it to train for your goal 6.2-miler, and with certain adjustments, you can also use it to prepare for everything from the 5-K to the marathon.

Four 10-K Training Universals

1. REST

Rest means no running—none. Give your muscles some serious R & R so all systems are primed for the next workout. Better 2 quality days and 2 of total rest than 4 days of mediocrity resulting from lingering fatigue. Rest days give you a mental break as well, so you'll come back feeling refreshed.

2. EASY RUNS

Easy means totally comfortable and controlled. If you're running with someone else, you should be able to converse easily. You'll likely feel as if you could go faster. Don't.

3. LONG RUNS

This is any steady run at or longer than race distance designed to enhance endurance, which enables you to run longer and longer and feel strong doing it. Find a weekly training partner for company. You'll have plenty of time to talk about anything that comes up.

4. SPEED

This means running in bursts at a distance shorter than the race—some at your race goal pace, some faster—which increases cardiovascular strength, biomechanical efficiency that translates into more miles per gallon, and the psychological toughness racing demands.

Beginner

You're a notch above novice. You've been running at least 6 months and maybe have done a 5-K or two. You run 3 to 5 miles 3 or 4 days a week, have done a little fast running when you felt like it, and now you want to enter—and finish—what you consider a real "distance race." If you're a beginner, your 10-K goal is less a personal record (PR) than an LDF (longest distance finished). You want to run the whole 6.2 miles, so you're going for endurance. "Basic aerobic strength is every runner's first need," says Sinclair. So you'll do most of your running at a steady, moderate pace. But we're also going to add a dash of speedwork into your endurance stew. This will put some added spring into your step, give you a brief taste of what it feels like to run a little faster, and hasten your segue to the intermediate level. Every week, in addition to steady running, you're going to do two extra things: aerobic intervals and gentle pickups.

Beginner 10-K Training Plan

WEEK	MON	TUES	WED	THURS	FRI	SAT	SUN	TOTAL
1	Rest	2 mi, 4 × 1:00 AI, 2 mi	3 mi or rest	4 mi + 3 strides	Rest	5 mi	Rest	13–20 mi
2	Rest	2 mi	3 mi or rest	4 mi + 3 strides	Rest	5.5 mi	3.5 mi	15–21 mi
3	Rest	2 mi, 4 × 1:30 AI, 2 mi	3 mi or rest	4.5 mi + 3 strides	Rest	6 mi	4 mi	18.5–22 mi
4	Rest	2 mi, 6 × 1:30 AI, 2 mi	3 mi or rest	4.5 mi + 3 strides	Rest	6.5 mi	4.5 mi	20–24 mi
5	Rest	2 mi, 4 × 2:00 AI, 2 mi	2 mi	Rest	2 mi + 2 strides	Rest	10-K race	

Stuff You Need to Know

AEROBIC INTERVALS (AI): Push the pace just a bit and breathe a little harder. Follow by slowly jogging until you feel rested enough to resume your regular tempo. Treat these runs like play. When you do them, try to re-create that feeling you had as a kid when you ran to the park and couldn't wait to get there.

STRIDES (S): Gradually pick up speed to about 90 percent effort; hold that for 60 yards, then decelerate. Walk to full recovery before you start the next one. Nothing big, nothing really stressful—just enough to let your body go, "Ah, so this is what it feels like to go fast."

Intermediate

You've been running a year or more, done some 5-Ks, maybe even a 10-K. But you always finish feeling like you could have or should have gone faster. You consider yourself mainly a recreational runner, but you still want to make a commitment to see how fast you can go. Here's the two-pronged approach that will move you to the cusp of competitive athlete.

First, you'll add miles to your endurance-building long run until it makes up

Intermediate 10-K Training Plan

WEEK	MON	TUES	WED	THURS	FRI	SAT	SUN	TOTAL
1	Rest	2 mi, 1 or 2 x tempo, 2 mi	4 mi	1 × 400 m PI, 1 × 800 m PI, 1 × 1200 m PI, 1 × 800 m PI, 1 × 400 m PI	Rest	4 mi, 4 × 100 m S	6–7 mi	23–24 mi
2	Rest	6 mi, incl 6:00 TUT	4 mi	1 × 1200 m PI, 2 × 800 m PI, 4 × 200 m PI, 4 × 200 m SI, 4 × 100 m S	Rest	4.5 mi, 5 × 100 m S	7–8 mi	29–30 mi
3	Rest	2 mi, 2 or 3 x tempo, 2 mi	4 mi	1 × 800 m PI, 1 × 1200 m PI, 1 × 800 m PI, 2 × 400 m SI, 4 × 200 m SI	Rest	5 mi, 6 × 100 m S	7–8 mi	29–30 mi
4	Rest	6–7 mi, incl 8:00 TUT	4 mi	1 × 1200 m PI, 1 × 800 m SI, 2 × 400 m SI, 2 × 200 m SI, 4 × 100 m S	Rest	5 mi, 6 × 100 m S	8–9 mi	30–32 mi
5	Rest	2 mi, 3 or 4 x tempo, 2 mi	4 mi	1 × 800 m SI, 4 × 400 m SI, 4 × 200 m SI, 1 × 800 m SI, 4 × 100 m S	Rest	6 mi, 6 × 100 m S	8–9 mi	31–32 mi
Taper	Rest	800 m SI, 2 × 200 m SI, 400 m SI, 2 × 200 m SI, 6 × 100 m S	4 mi, 4 × 200 m SI, 4 × 100 m S	Rest	3 mi easy, 3 × 100 m S	10-K race		

30 percent of your weekly mileage. Second, you'll now do a substantial amount of tempo running. This will significantly improve your endurance and running efficiency in just 6 weeks. So your tempo work will include weekly "10-10s," along with intervals and uphill running, all of which strengthen your running muscles, heart, and related aerobic systems.

Oh, one more thing: Running fast requires effort—and some discomfort. Still, be conservative. If you can't maintain the same pace throughout a given workout or your body shrieks "*No mas!*" then call it a day. And maybe adjust your pace next time.

Stuff You Need to Know

PACE INTERVALS (PI): Run at 10-K goal pace to improve efficiency and stamina and to give you the feel of your race pace. With pace and speed intervals (below), jog half the interval distance to recover. For 10:00 (10-minute) goal pace (a 1:02:06 10-K), run 2:30 (for 400 meters), 5:00 (800 meters), 7:30 (1200 meters). For 9:00 pace (55:53), run 2:15 (400 meters), 4:30 (800 meters), 6:45 (1200 meters). For 8:00 pace (49:40), run 2:00 (400 meters), 4:00 (800 meters), 6:00 (1200 meters).

SPEED INTERVALS (SI): Run these at 30 seconds per mile faster than goal pace. For 10:00 pace, run 2:22 (400 meters), 4:44 (800 meters), 7:06 (1200 meters). For 9:00 pace, run 2:08 (400 meters), 4:16 (800 meters), 6:24 (1200 meters). For 8:00 pace, run 1:53 (400 meters), 3:45 (800 meters), 5:38 (1200 meters).

TEMPO: Run 10-minute tempo repeats at 30 seconds per mile slower than 10-K goal pace; follow each with a 3- to 5-minute slow jog.

TOTAL UPHILL TIME (TUT): Run repetitions up the same hill, or work the uphill sections of a road or trail course.

STRIDES (S): Gradually pick up speed to about 90 percent effort; hold that for 60 yards, then decelerate. Walk to full recovery before you start the next one. Nothing big, nothing really stressful—just enough to let your body go, "Ah, so this is what it feels like to go fast."

Advanced

You've been a serious runner for several years and have run many races—perhaps even a marathon. You're familiar with fartleks and intervals and can run comfortably for an hour-plus. Now you want a breakthrough time—and you're willing to put in a rigorous 6 weeks to achieve it.

This plan is a 6-week diet of quick stuff—medium long on Tuesdays, short and swift on Thursdays. And to make sure you maintain your vital aerobic base, you'll be logging solid mileage as well.

Advanced 10-K Training Plan

WEEK	MON	TUES	WED	THURS	FRI	SAT	SUN	TOTAL
1	Rest	2 × 1200 PI, 2 × 800 PI, 4 × 400 PI, 6 × 100 S	4–6 mi	2 × 800 SI, 4 × 400 SI, 4 × 200 SI, 4 × 100 S	Rest or 3–4 mi easy	4–6 mi, 6 × 100 S	8–10 mi	32–42 mi
2	Rest	2 × 1200 PI, 1 × 800 SI, 1 × 400 SI, 1 × 200 SI, 6 × 100 S	4–6 mi	4 × 200 SI, 4 LS, 4 × 100 S	Rest or 3–4 mi easy	5–7 mi, 6 × 100 S	8–10 mi	32–42 mi
3	Rest	2 × 1 mi PI, 1 × 1200 PI, 1 × 800 SI, 1 × 400 SI, 6 × 100 S	4–6 mi	4 × 200 SI, 4 LS, 4 × 200 SI, 4 × 100 S	Rest or 3–4 mi easy	5–7 mi	9–11 mi	33–43 mi
4	Rest	2 × 1200 PI, 1 × 800 SI, 1 × 400 SI, 1 × 200 SI, 6 × 100 S	4–6 mi	5–7 LS, 6 × 100 S	Rest or 3–4 mi easy	5–7 mi, 6 × 100 S	9–11 mi	33–44 mi
5	Rest	2 × 400 SI, 1 × 800 SI, 1 × 200 SI, 1 × 800 SI, 6 × 100 S	4–6 mi	6–8 mi	Rest or 3–4 mi easy	5–7 mi, 6 × 100 S	10–12 mi	34–46 mi
Taper	Rest	1 × 1200 PI, 1 × 800 S, 2 × 400 SI, 4 × 100 S	Rest	4 × 200 SI, 4 × 100 S, 4 × 200 SI, 4 × 100 S	Rest	3 mi easy, 3 × 100 S	10-K race	

Stuff You Need to Know

PACE INTERVALS (PI): For both pace and speed intervals, run 2 miles easy, plus four 100-meter strides before each session and 2 miles easy afterward. For 8:00 (8-minute) goal pace (49:40 finishing time), run 2:00 (for 400 meters), 4:00 (800 meters), 6:00 (1200 meters). For 7:00 pace (43:28), run 0:53 (200 meters), 1:45 (400 meters), 3:30 (800 meters), 5:15 (1200 meters). For 6:00 pace (37:15), run 0:45 (200 meters), 1:30 (400 meters), 4:30 (1200 meters). Recovery is a 1-minute jog (after 400-meter reps), 2:00 (800 meters), and 3:00 (1200 meters).

SPEED INTERVALS (SI): For 8:00 pace, run 1:53 (400 meters), 3:45 (800 meters) 5:38 (1200 meters). For 7:00 pace, run 0:49 (200 meters), 1:38 (400 meters), 4:53 (1200 meters). For 6:00 pace, run 0:41 (200 meters), 1:22 (400 meters), 2:44 (800 meters), 4:08 (1200 meters).

LACTATE SESSIONS (LS): LS training involves running about as fast as you can for 1 minute, followed by 3 to 4 minutes of slow jogging.

STRIDES (S): Over 100 meters, gradually accelerate to about 90 percent of all-out, hold it there for 5 seconds, and then smoothly decelerate. Walk to full recovery after each. Strides aren't meant to tire you out—just the opposite. They'll add zip to your legs.

CHART YOUR PROGRESS

Keep an even pace, calculate your average pace after a race, and improve your time the chart below. Find your time per mile in the vertical column on the left and read across the chart horizontally to find your projected finish time.

TIME/MILE	2 MI	5-K/3.1 MI	4 MI	5 MI	10-K/6.2 MI	12-K/7.46 MI
5:45	11:30	17:52	23:00	28:45	35:44	42:52
6:00	12:00	18:39	24:00	30:00	37:17	44:44
6:15	12:30	19:25	25:00	31:15	38:50	46:36
6:30	13:00	20:12	26:00	32:30	40:23	48:28
6:45	13:30	20:58	27:00	33:45	41:57	50:20
7:00	14:00	21:45	28:00	35:00	43:30	52:12
7:15	14:30	22:32	29:00	36:15	45:03	54:03
7:30	15:00	23:18	30:00	37:30	46:36	55:55
7:45	15:30	24:05	31:00	38:45	48:10	57:47
8:00	16:00	24:51	32:00	40:00	49:43	59:39
8:15	16:30	25:38	33:00	41:15	51:16	1:01:31
8:30	17:00	26:25	34:00	42:30	52:49	1:03:23
8:45	17:30	27:11	35:00	43:45	54:22	1:05:14
9:00	18:00	27:58	36:00	45:00	55:56	1:07:06
9:15	18:30	28:44	37:00	46:15	57:29	1:08:58
9:30	19:00	29:31	38:00	47:30	59:02	1:10:50
9:45	19:30	30:18	39:00	48:45	1:00:35	1:12:42
10:00	20:00	31:04	40:00	50:00	1:02:08	1:14:34
10:30	21:00	32:37	42:00	52:30	1:05:15	1:18:17
11:00	22:00	34:11	44:00	55:00	1:08:21	1:22:01
11:30	23:00	35:44	46:00	57:30	1:11:28	1:25:45
12:00	24:00	37:17	48:00	1:00:00	1:14:34	1:29:28
12:30	25:00	38:50	50:00	1:02:30	1:17:41	1:33:12
13:00	26:00	40:23	52:00	1:05:00	1:20:47	1:36:56

15-K/9.3 MI	10 MI	20-K/12.34 MI	HALF-MARATHON/13.1 MI	15 MI	20 MI	MARATHON/26.2 MI
53:36	57:30	1:11:27	1:15:23	1:26:15	1:55:00	2:30:46
55:56	1:00:00	1:14:34	1:18:39	1:30:00	2:00:00	2:37:19
58:15	1:02:30	1:17:40	1:21:56	1:33:45	2:05:00	2:43:52
1:00:35	1:05:00	1:20:47	1:25:13	1:37:30	2:10:00	2:50:25
1:02:55	1:07:30	1:23:53	1:28:29	1:41:15	2:15:00	2:56:59
1:05:15	1:10:00	1:26:59	1:31:46	1:45:00	2:20:00	3:03:32
1:07:35	1:12:30	1:30:06	1:35:02	1:48:45	2:25:00	3:10:05
1:09:54	1:15:00	1:33:12	1:38:19	1:52:30	2:30:00	3:16:39
1:12:14	1:17:30	1:36:19	1:41:36	1:56:15	2:35:00	3:23:12
1:14:34	1:20:00	1:39:25	1:44:52	2:00:00	2:40:00	3:29:45
1:16:54	1:22:30	1:42:31	1:48:09	2:03:45	2:45:00	3:36:18
1:19:14	1:25:00	1:45:38	1:51:26	2:07:30	2:50:00	3:42:52
1:21:34	1:27:30	1:48:44	1:54:42	2:11:15	2:55:00	3:49:25
1:23:53	1:30:00	1:51:51	1:57:59	2:15:00	3:00:00	3:55:58
1:26:13	1:32:30	1:54:57	2:01:15	2:18:45	3:5:00	4:02:32
1:28:33	1:35:00	1:58:03	2:04:32	2:22:30	3:10:00	4:09:05
1:30:53	1:37:30	2:01:10	2:07:49	2:26:15	3:15:00	4:15:38
1:33:13	1:40:00	2:04:16	2:11:05	2:30:00	3:20:00	4:22:11
1:37:52	1:45:00	2:10:29	2:17:39	2:37:30	3:30:00	4:35:18
1:42:32	1:50:00	2:16:42	2:24:12	2:45:00	3:40:00	4:48:25
1:47:11	1:55:00	2:22:55	2:30:45	2:52:30	3:50:00	5:01:31
1:51:51	2:00:00	2:29:07	2:37:18	3:00:00	4:00:00	5:14:38
1:56:31	2:05:00	2:35:20	2:43:52	3:07:30	4:10:00	5:27:44
2:01:10	2:10:00	2:41:33	2:50:25	3:15:00	4:20:00	5:40:51

NUTRITION
26 BEST FOODS FOR RUNNERS

Food is fuel. But it's also something that has to satisfy your tastebuds or you're not going to eat it. And what good will that do you. Below you'll find the absolute best foods for runners—and there's nothing on the list that'll make you gag. Start with the Magnificent Six, powerhouse foods that should be every runner's staples. They will secure your continued good health and power your running.

The Magnificent Six

1. EGGS: One egg fulfills about 10 percent of your daily protein needs. Egg protein is a complete protein, which means it contains all the crucial amino acids your hard-working muscles need to promote recovery.

2. SALMON: Besides being an excellent source of protein, salmon is one of the best sources of omega-3 fats. These fats help balance the body's inflammation response, which has been linked to many chronic diseases.

3. SWEET POTATOES: Sweet potatoes are a good source of vitamins A and C, potassium, iron, as well as the trace minerals manganese and copper, which are crucial for healthy muscle function.

4. ORANGES: Eat enough oranges and you may feel less achy after hard workouts. Oranges supply more than 100 percent of the Daily Value for the antioxidant vitamin C, which has been linked to alleviating muscle soreness.

5. CANNED BLACK BEANS: Black beans and other legumes are low glycemic index (GI) foods, meaning the carb is released slowly into the body. Low GI foods can help control blood sugar and may enhance performance because of their steady release of energy.

6. MIXED SALAD GREENS: They're loaded with phytonutrients that may fend off age-related diseases, like Alzheimer's, heart disease, and diabetes. These nutrients also act as antioxidants, warding off muscle damage brought on by tough workouts.

Five Prerun Snacks That Are Ready to Eat Now

7. HANDFUL OF LOW-FIBER CEREAL
8. A BAGEL WITH HONEY OR JELLY
9. A FEW GRAHAM CRACKERS WITH A TEASPOON OF HONEY
10. BANANA AND A FEW NUTS OR TEASPOON OF PEANUT BUTTER
11. CUP OF FAT-FREE YOGURT

The Runner's Pantry

Stock up on these essentials to ensure an at-the-ready supply of basics on which to build run-fueling meals and snacks.

12. **BULGUR:** This grain cooks fast and makes great salads and breakfast cereal

13. **BROWN AND WILD RICE:** provide variety to your grains and also a good source of fiber

14. **OLIVE OIL:** Choose extra-virgin, which is less processed than other types. Its monounsaturated fat has been shown to lower "bad" cholesterol and improve heart health. Drizzle it over salads, potatoes, and pasta.

15. **FRESH HERBS:** They elevate other healthy foods from so-so to sensational. Mint freshens up salads, potatoes, even beverages. Basil enhances beans and tomatoes. Rub rosemary into chicken or salmon.

16. **LONG-KEEPING VEGETABLES AND FRUITS:** Carrots, kale, zucchini, and lemons keep for a week or more; potatoes, onions, and garlic last even longer. Buy frozen spinach and corn to enjoy these fast-fading veggies anytime.

17. **CANNED TOMATOES:** Indispensable for making superfast sauces for pasta or chicken.

18. **DRIED FRUIT AND NUTS:** Having these healthy snacks on hand keeps you from overeating at meals. They also make tasty add-ins for salads and grain-based side dishes.

Carb Favorites

19. **BEER:** Indulge by downing a stout or porter instead of lighter, amber ales: These dark beers contain a few more calories per bottle, but they also have far more antioxidants from the wheat and other grains used to make them.

20. **PASTA:** Go for the whole grain variety.

The Healthiest Chocolate for Runners

21. **DARK CHOCOLATE:** Research indicates that flavanols, the compounds found in cocoa, have antioxidant properties that help mop up the damage done by free radicals. These same compounds also relax artery walls and keep blood platelets from sticking to your arteries, thus reducing your chance of heart disease.

22. **LOW-FAT CHOCOLATE MILK:** It provides an ideal mix of quick-digesting carbs and protein to promote recovery. Plus, the chocolate helps satisfy occasional sweet cravings.

Eat This Stuff in Season

Max out flavor and nutritional value by eating prime-time produce.

23. **BEETS:** A 2009 study found that cyclists who drank 500 milliliters of beet juice exercised 16 percent longer than those who drank a placebo.

24. **PUMPKIN SEEDS:** Muscle-fueling minerals. Rich in magnesium and iron, protein, vitamin K, and heart-healthy mono- and polyunsaturated fats—all for less than 200 calories per $\frac{1}{2}$ cup.

25. **SPAGHETTI SQUASH:** A nutritious noodle. One cup contains 42 calories and two grams of fiber; it's also a good source of vitamin B_6, vitamin C, manganese, potassium, and iron.

26. **APPLES:** Apples are among the best food sources of quercetin, an antioxidant that can boost endurance.

FUELING RULES

Wondering what to eat and drink, and how much? Here are four basic rules to follow while training for your first 5-K.

Rule #1 Have a drink

Getting enough fluids is key, as being a little dehydrated can affect your performance. Try to get 16 ounces of water about an hour before your run, and rehydrate afterward. And be sure to stay hydrated throughout the day. Drink half your body weight in ounces. So if you weigh 150 pounds, drink 75 ounces of water per day. If you weigh 100 pounds, have 50 ounces.

Rule #2 Emphasize carbohydrates

Carbs are a runner's most important energy source. Aim for a 50-25-25 eating plan, where 50 percent of your calories come from carbohydrates, 25 percent from protein, and 25 percent from fat. With half of your calories coming from carbohydrates, this will provide you with plenty of readily available fuel for your runs. Proteins and fats will help you feel full longer and give you important nutrients you need.

Rule #3 Eat real food

When you're in training, it's best to eat a variety of healthful foods throughout the day, including fruits, vegetables, whole grains, low-fat dairy products such as milk and cheese, and lean meats. Don't over-rely on so-called "performance foods," such as energy bars, gels, sports drinks, and the like. These are all fine—they have their uses, especially before, during, and after running—but you won't need them while ramping up for a 5-K.

Rule #4 Keep it simple

You need to be energized on the run, but you don't want to be sidelined with stomach issues. Don't try any new foods before a run or your race. In the hours before you run, have carbs like bananas, low-fiber cereal, bagels, yogurt, or oatmeal. Stay away from too much protein, fat, or fiber, which can cause stomach distress on the road.

The Drink Menu

Does your running call for water, or something stronger? Here's how to choose the best beverage.

	WHAT IT IS	WHEN IT'S RIGHT
Water	Tap or bottled, water provides calorie-free hydration—a boon for those watching their weight.	On runs 30 minutes and shorter, since your stored energy can meet the workout's demands. It's best for anytime hydration: Drink water during and between meals to replace fluid lost during workouts.
Enhanced Water	These low-calorie drinks often contain a trace of sweetener, vitamins and minerals—but not enough to boost running performance.	When plain water seems boring.
Sports Drinks	Their low carbohydrate concentration (six to eight percent, or 14 to 20 grams of carbs per serving) replenish spent stores 30 percent faster than with plain water. They also contain sodium and potassium, electrolytes that are lost through sweat and important for fluid retention.	Before, during, and after runs longer than 30 minutes. Don't balk at the calories: Research indicates that consuming carbs during exercise may suppress appetite later.
Endurance Sports Drinks	These formulas have the same amount of carbs as regular sports drinks, but boast an extra dose of electrolytes such as potassium (and twice the sodium of sports brews).	Best for distance runners: Drink these during workouts or races lasting two hours or more. Also good for runners who sweat a lot or tend to cramp during long runs.
Energy Drinks	Caffeine and sugar provide the advertised "energy." Containing 110 to 160 sugar calories per eight-ounce serving, their dense carb content slows fluid absorption and can cause stomach upset. Other stimulants (such as guarana, ginseng, and taurine) may increase blood pressure and make you feel shaky, especially on an empty stomach.	For supplemental fluids and carbs before and after a run, and when calories aren't a concern.
Recovery Drinks	These potions combine carbs with protein, which facilitates muscle repair and improves the body's ability to replenish its glycogen stores. Most contain 30 to 60 grams of carbs and seven to 15 grams of protein (for a four-to-one ratio).	After a race or tough workout, especially when the exertion makes solid foods unappetizing.
Juice and Soft Drinks	They'll hydrate you, but their dense carb concentration (10 to 14 percent) slows fluid absorption in the intestines and can cause stomach distress in some runners when sipped during exercise. 100 percent real fruit juices contain vitamins; soda delivers no nutritional value.	At snack time, or before a run.

A Perfect Day for Weight Loss

Shedding pounds doesn't require starvation. Here's a delicious 24-hour menu.

RUNNER: 35 years old, 150 pounds

LIFESTYLE: Sedentary desk job

EXERCISE: Runs about 20 miles per week at a nine-minute per-mile pace; strength trains about two hours per week

MAINTENANCE CALORIE NEEDS: 2,387 calories per day

GOAL CALORIE INTAKE: 2,029 calories (15 percent reduction)

Breakfast

2 slices whole-grain toast; 2 teaspoons almond butter; 1 kiwi; 1 hard-boiled egg

A breakfast containing a balanced mix of carbs, protein, and healthy fats prevents over-eating during the day.

Morning snack

1 cup plain low-fat yogurt; $\frac{1}{2}$ cup raspberries; 1 ounce sunflower seeds

Have a midmorning snack to hold off hunger while providing energy for your lunchtime workout.

Lunch workout

30- to 40-minute interval run

Postrun

1 cup low-fat chocolate milk

It provides an ideal mix of quick-digesting carbs and protein to promote recovery. Plus, the chocolate helps satisfy occasional sweet cravings.

Lunch

1 serving (2 cups) whole-wheat pasta with kidney beans and veggies; 1 medium apple

Make the pasta for dinner the night before and pack the leftovers for lunch.

Dinner
4 ounces chicken breast; 1 cup cooked quinoa; 1 cup multicolored salad; $^1/_3$ of an avocado; 1 tablespoon extra-virgin-olive-oil and-vinegar dressing

The healthy fat in olive oil and avocado slows digestion (keeping you satisfied) and boosts the absorption of antioxidants in veggies.

Evening snack
3 cups air-popped popcorn

When air-popped, it makes a tasty and healthy whole-grain, low-calorie snack for the evening.

Calories: 1,991 • carbs: 252 g • fiber: 47 g • protein: 113 g • fat: 67 g

Top Ways to Lose Weight

Try these runners' diet strategies to shed pounds while you're in training

Ditch diet foods

They may seem like a bargain, calorie-wise, but most diet foods are too low in carbs, fiber, or protein to keep you satisfied. The result? You eat more of other foods than you normally would. Opt for real foods, but limit portions.

Get your Zs

Research suggests that people who skimp on sleep eat more snacks and weigh more than those who are well-rested. Without enough sleep, your energy levels, immune system, and mood all take a hit. Power down earlier at night so you can run feeling supercharged.

Eat colorfully

Pale foods (such as pasta and potatoes) have their place on runners' plates, but a rainbow-hued diet includes berries, carrots, broccoli, tomatoes—fruits and vegetables that are low in calories but high in run-fueling nutrients.

Build muscle

Even at rest, muscle uses oxygen and thus burns calories, so add strength training to your weekly regimen.

Challenge yourself

The more routine your running becomes, the fewer calories you'll burn. Bust out of the rut by boosting your intensity and doing different types of workouts (like a weekly long run or a day of cross-training) to challenge your body and burn more calories.

Embrace fats

Fat keeps you satisfied and prevents your blood sugar from plummeting, which keeps you from overeating later in the day. Choose unsaturated fats to help lower LDL and reduce your risk of heart disease: Some research suggests that a diet rich in monounsaturated fats can also help prevent weight gain.

Control emotional eating

Reaching for the cookie jar when you're feeling blue puts on unwanted pounds. Learn to separate comfort cravings from genuine hunger: If a healthy food choice doesn't satisfy your urge, you're seeking mood-lifters, not fuel.

Get a scale

People who weigh themselves daily or weekly lose more weight (and keep it off) than dieters who rarely step on a scale.

Go slow

Slashing calories and working out like a machine gets old, fast—and once you abandon the too-ambitious routine, it's easy to regain any weight you lost. Set modest goals—like slashing 300 calories per day—that require small changes, not whole-life overhauls.

Eat breakfast

Within 2 hours of waking, eat a breakfast that includes carbohydrates (for energy) and protein (for satiety). That way, you'll be less susceptible to a midmorning doughnut indulgence.

INJURY PREVENTION
FIVE TIPS FOR PAIN-FREE RUNNIING

I t's difficult to be a happy runner when your illiotibial band is inflamed and taking your name in vain with every stride. Stay energized and healthy while training by keeping these key strategies in mind.

Build Up Gradually

Stick to the plan, and build your miles gradually over the course of the plan. This ensures that your bones, muscles, and ligaments have time to adjust to the increased workload—without injury.

Listen to Your Body

Pay attention to warning signs such as recurring pain or fatigue that doesn't go away even with sleep. It's also important to pay attention to what's working for you. If you feel energized after eating a particular prerun snack, for instance, remember it and try it again.

Watch Your Step

Don't assume a driver sees you. In fact, assume that a driver can't see you. Run against traffic so you can see any sudden moves an advancing motorist may make. At a stop sign or light, wait for the driver to wave you through—then acknowledge with your own wave. Always be prepared to jump onto the sidewalk or shoulder of the road.

Get Some Sleep

Sleep is critical for muscle repair and regeneration. Keep your bedroom dark, cool, and quiet. Also, consider blackout window shades, and avoid using a TV, laptop, or smart phone 30 minutes before bedtime.

Respond to Pain

It's normal to feel some muscle soreness after a run, but if the pain persists for more than a day, or persists or worsens while you are running, stop and see a doctor. Cross-train in the meantime with cycling, swimming, or riding a stationary bike or elliptical.

BEAT THE HEAT
RUN THIS WAY WHEN IT'S HOT OUTSIDE

Even if you don't push the pace, running in hot weather makes your body work harder. It can be uncomfortable, and downright dangerous, if you don't take the proper precautions. But that doesn't mean your marathon and half-marathon training has to take a siesta for June, July, and August. Here are some tips for beating the heat to keep your training on track.

Head Out Early or Late

Even in the worst heat wave, temps cools off significantly by dawn. Get your run done then, and you'll feel good about it all day. Can't fit it in? Wait until evening, when the power has gone out of the sun—just don't do it so late that it keeps you from getting to sleep.

Adjust Your Expectations

Every 5° rise in temperature above 60°F can slow your pace up to 20 to 30 seconds per mile. If you have a speed session scheduled and temperatures are soaring, reschedule it and run easy instead. Start your run 30 seconds per mile slower than your normal training pace.

Prevent Sunburn

To lower your risk, avoid the sun between 10 a.m. and 4 p.m., wear a hat, run in the shade, and wear sunscreen with an SPF of 30 with broad spectrum protection. Apply the sunscreen 20 minutes before you head out, so your skin has time to absorb it. Reapply sunscreen every hour.

Drink Early and Often

Top off your fluid stores with 16 ounces of sports drink an hour before you head out. Then toss down five to eight ounces of sports drink about every 20 minutes while running. Sports drinks beat water because they contain electrolytes, which replace the electrolytes you lose in sweat, and they taste good, so it's easy to drink more.

Take the Sweat Test

Because sweat rates vary enormously, you can get an idea of your own sweat rate by weighing yourself naked before and after a couple of runs. If, for example, you lose one pound during a 40-minute run, it means you sweated about 16 ounces of fluid. Going forward you can then try to replenish your fluids at a rate of about 16 ounces per 40 minutes of running. Take the sweat test in as many different conditions as possible.

Watch for Blisters

Summer is prime time for blisters, which are caused by friction, excessive moisture (from sweaty feet), or shoes that don't fit right. Putting Vaseline, sports lube, and bandages over blister-prone spots may also help. Ignore blisters smaller than 5 millimeters (the size of a pencil eraser). But pop the bigger ones. With a sterile needle, prick the side of the blister and drain it. Don't remove the top of the blister. Instead, cover it with an antibiotic ointment and moleskin or a bandage.

Avoid Chafing

Skin-to-skin and skin-to-clothing rubbing can cause a red, raw rash that can bleed, sting, and make you yelp during your postrun shower. Moisture and salt (from sweat) make it worse. To prevent chafing, wear moisture-wicking, seamless, tagless gear. Apply Vaseline, sports lube, Band-Aids, or NipGuards before you run. To treat it, wash the area with soap and water, apply an antibacterial ointment, and cover with a bandage.

Get Used to It

Give yourself up to 14 days to acclimatize to hot weather, gradually increasing the length and intensity of your training. In that time, your body will learn to decrease your heart rate, decrease your core body temperature, and increase your sweat rate. Do your main workouts before 10 a.m. or after 6 p.m., and start with a 15-to 20-minute light run or walk in the heat of the day. Increase the length of your hot workouts by five to 10 minutes over two weeks. Allow even more time to adjust to humid environments.

Look for Grass and Shade

It's always hotter in cities than in surrounding areas because asphalt and concrete retain heat. If you must run in an urban or even a suburban area, look for shade.

DON'T STALL IN WINTER
RUN THIS WAY WHEN IT'S FRIGID

Between the wind, the snow, the dark, and the chilly temperatures, winter can blow a flurry of new obstacles into your running routine. (And then there are those pesky kids with the snowballs.) Here are some tips to help you plow through the season and keep your training on track.

Watch Your Step

You'll get better traction on snow that's been packed down (fresh powder can cover up ice patches). Wear a scarf or a ski mask to warm up the cold air so it doesn't hurt your lungs. Run on the street if it's been plowed (as long as it's safe from traffic), and watch out for black ice. Run on the sidewalk if it's clear of ice. Find a well-lit route; slow your pace.

Run Midday

If possible, run during the light hours, the warmest time of day. The little dose of sunshine will help, and much of the ice will be melted.

Start into the Wind

Start an out-and-back run in to the wind, so you have it blowing at your back on your way home. You'll avoid getting chilled by the wind after you've been sweating.

Shorten Your Stride

When running on ice or snow, shorten your stride to help prevent slipping and falling. Focus on getting in time rather than pace or distance on challenging weather days. Use products like Yak Trax to reduce the risk of falling.

Warm Up and Cool Down

When it's cold out, your ligaments, tendons, and muscles take longer to loosen up, so extend your warmup. You might walk for 5 minutes, then spend 5 to 10 minutes alternating between walking and jogging as you ramp up to your target pace. When it's below freezing, try part of your warmup indoors. Start your run on a treadmill, then head out once your legs feel ready but before you start sweating. After the run, keep your cooldown brief to avoid getting too chilled: Slow your pace for 3 to 4 minutes, then go inside. Take extra layers off and keep moving (walking on a treadmill, or just around your house) for another 5 to 10 minutes before hitting the shower.

Layer Up

Dress in thin, light, wick-away layers that you can add or take off to suit your temperature. Make sure you have a running gear that blocks the wind and base layers that wick sweat away from your skin; don't go out without gloves, mittens, and a hat or headband to cover your head. Dress for 15°F to 20°F warmer. You should feel slightly chilled when you walk out the door. As you warm up and your body temperature starts to increase, you'll feel better. You want to reduce the risk of overheating and sweating excessively. Use the *Runner's World* "What Should I Wear" tool at runnersworld.com/tools. It will help you decide what to wear in all kinds of weather.

Defrost

Damp clothes increase heat loss. As soon as possible postrun, change into fleeces and sweats.

Find Safety in Numbers

With the dark and the ice, it's a great time to run with a buddy or join a running group. You'll have a built in reason to get out the door, and a friend to chat with along the way.

See and Be Seen

If you run in the dark hours, wear a reflective vest, a headlamp, or flashing lights so you're seen in traffic. In snowy weather, wear bright clothing. Run with ID just in case.

Take It Inside

If the roads are covered with ice, take it to the treadmill. Find hillwork, speed sessions, and long runs all for the mill on this page, plus reviews of the latest models here. If you can't stand the mill, cross-train on the bike or elliptical trainer for the same amount of time you'd spend running.

Set a Small Goal

There is nothing more motivating than to train for a race or goal. Set a goal to run a 5-K, half-marathon, or reach a number of miles every month! You'll have instant motivation in knowing you have to train for the race or hit your target mileage. Reward yourself with a treat—like new running gear—when you reach your goal. To find an event near you, check out our race finder at runnersworld .com/racefinder.

Be Flexible

In order to avoid missing workouts, always have a plan B. If you're usually a morning runner, be willing to run in the afternoon instead. If the street is an ice rink, head to the gym. Better to reframe your workout rather than ditch it. When you run, you feel good, and you keep at it. When you don't run, you start to feel stressed, which can cause a cascade of hormonal changes that can result in decreased motivation, fatigue, anxiety, and depression. Even if you can just get a 20-minute workout in, you'll feel better.

RESOURCES
GREAT READS

The Great Grete Waitz

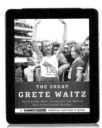

In *The Great Grete Waitz, Runner's World* has published the magazine's first e-book original, a moving tribute to the humble marathon legend who changed the landscape of running forever. The editors of the magazine have gathered a collection of the best stories about Grete from the last 30 years, providing a revealing glimpse into the "quiet queen" who won the New York City Marathon an astounding nine times, helping to turn the event into a worldwide phenomenon. *The Great Grete Waitz* is an unforgettable, across-the-decades portrait of a truly pioneering spirit who changed the sport of running forever.

Runner's World Complete Book of Running: Everything You Need to Know to Run for Fun, Fitness, and Competition
Edited by Amby Burfoot, editor-at-large, *Runner's World*, and winner of the 1968 Boston Marathon

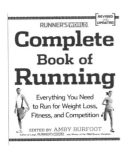

Inside *Runner's World Complete Book of Running* are all the secrets of running that beginner and veteran runners alike will ever need. With all-new photos and a fresh design, this revised edition has the advice—both timeless and cutting-edge—that is guaranteed to maximize any runner's performance and enjoyment of the sport.

Runner's World Essential Guides: Fast Fuel

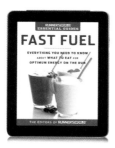

What should I eat? The question dogs all of us on a daily basis, but it's perhaps most vexing for runners, who rely on food to fuel their workouts and feel good. Most runners take in lots of calories and nutrients in the form of energy bars, nutrient-enhanced drinks, and fortified packaged foods. The problem is, "real" foods—fruits, vegetables, whole grains, and lean meats—are better for you than fortified products are. That's because there's more to a carrot or a sweet potato than just vitamin A. Within the body, vitamins, minerals, and other essential nutrients work together with literally thousands of other compounds, such as color components in fruits and vegetables, special starches and fibers in whole grains, and unique fats in seeds, nuts, and dairy. And it's the whole package that promotes good health and peak athletic performance.

Of course, protein bars and calcium-fortified juices seem like a convenient way to take in all of the nutrients every runner needs daily. But getting them—and more—from real food is preferable, and it's easy. *Runner's World Essential Guides: Fast Fuel* shows you exactly how. The world's foremost authorities on running have collected the best information, tips, and advice about eating on the run. This indispensable guide covers everything from eating for optimum energy to cooking simple, healthy meals to snacking smart and shopping for the best of the best foods to store in your pantry and fridge.

The Runner's World Essential Guides: Fast Fuel contains everything you need to know about eating right to feel better, run stronger, and recover faster.

Runner's World Essential Guides: Weight Loss

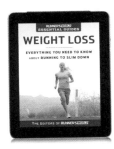

The miles you log are great for keeping you fit, healthy, and happy, and they help you to maintain your weight. But weight *loss* is a different story. Because you run, you may think you can eat whatever you want and still drop pounds. Unfortunately, that's not true. Running is only half the equation. You have to look hard at what and how you eat, too. Conventional dieting wisdom tends to leave runners hungry, tired, and overweight.

Let *Runner's World Essential Guides: Weight Loss* lead you through the minefield of dieting by showing you everything you need to know to shed pounds without losing steam on the run. The editors of *Runner's World,* the world's foremost authorities on running, have collected the best information about weight loss on the run, answering questions such as: What are the eight Golden Rules of weight loss? What should you eat to boost your metabolism? What are the best foods to eat for breakfast, lunch, and dinner to optimize weight loss? Weight-loss myths are debunked, and you'll get simple ideas for pre- and post-workout snacks as well as delicious, ridiculously easy-to-make recipes like a healthy hamburger and an angel food cake. With this guide, you'll have the fuel you need to run and the knowledge you need to shed pounds and keep them off once and for all!

Run!
by Dean Karnazes

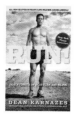

In this *New York Times* bestseller, *Runner's World* contributing editor Dean Karnazes chronicles his unbelievable exploits and explorations in gripping detail. From the downright hilarious to the truly profound, the stories in *Run!* provide readers with the ultimate escape, offering a rare glimpse into the mind-set and motivation of an extreme athlete. Karnazes addresses the pain and perseverance and also charts his emotional state as he pushes the edges of human achievement. The result is a romp with running at its heart and soul. The tales of friendships he's cultivated on adventures around the world will inspire readers whether they run great distances, modest distances, or not at all.

Run Your Butt Off!
by Sarah Lorge Butler with Leslie Bonci, MPH, RD, and Budd Coates, MS, the *Runner's World* running coach

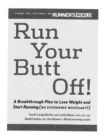

Shed unwanted pounds and keep them off once and for all with *Run Your Butt Off!*—a back-to-basics, test panel–approved weight-loss plan and beginner running program that yields sustainable, healthy results. The *Run Your Butt Off!* program is founded on the simple concept that, in order to lose weight, calories burned must exceed calories consumed. With this program, you'll learn to burn fat from both sides of the weight-loss equation—the calories in and the calories out—at the same time. *Run Your Butt Off!* will make you fitter, stronger, and leaner.

Runner's World Run Less Run Faster
by Bill Pierce, Scott Murr, and Ray Moss

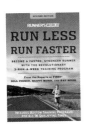

Improve your race times while training less with the revolutionary Furman Institute of Running and Scientific Training (FIRST) program. FIRST's philosophy limits overtraining and burnout and cuts the risk of injury—while producing faster race times. The key feature is the "three plus two" weekly program: three quality runs to improve endurance and leg speed, plus two aerobic cross-training workouts. With training plans for 5-K, 10-K, half-marathon, and marathon distances, plus tips for goal-setting, recovery, injury rehab and prevention, strength training, and nutrition, this program will change the way you train.

Runner's World Complete Book of Women's Running: The Best Advice to Get Started, Stay Motivated, Lose Weight, Run Injury-Free, Be Safe, and Train for Any Distance
by Dagny Scott Barrios

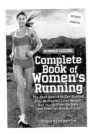

Women are redefining running. They run to get in shape, lose weight, relax, manage stress, and for the sheer enjoyment of the sport. Packed with how-to advice, tips, and strategies, the *Runner's World Complete Book of Women's Running* brings the sport to life through the personal accounts and testimonials of women runners of all ages and abilities. It's a must-read for every woman who runs.

Going Long: Legends, Oddballs, Comebacks, & Adventures
The Best Stories from Runner's World
edited by David Willey

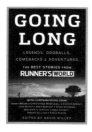

For more than 40 years, *Runner's World* magazine has been the world's leading authority on running—bringing its readers the latest advice on training and nutrition and some of the most compelling sports narratives ever told. The magazine captures the minds, hearts, and emotions of its readers every month. Now, the editors of *Runner's World* have gathered powerful tales into *Going Long,* a book with more than 40 stories that transcend the sport of running to reach any reader with an appetite for drama, inspiration, and a glimpse into the human condition.

Marathon (4th Edition)
by Hal Higdon

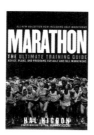

Longtime *Runner's World* contributor Hal Higdon presents a completely revised and expanded edition of his classic guide to taking the guesswork out of preparing for a marathon, whether it's a reader's first or fiftieth. At the core of the book is Higdon's clear and essential information on training, injury prevention, and nutrition. Exclusive new material includes training plans for half-marathons and vital tips for women runners. Higdon's book is the most successful marathon book ever for marathon runners for a good reason: It works. Whether your goal is to finish, set a personal record, or qualify for the Boston Marathon, Higdon will show you how.

My Life on the Run: The Wit, Wisdom, and Insights of a Road Racing Icon
by Bart Yasso with Kathleen Parrish

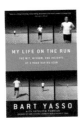

The revered *Runner's World* chief running officer offers a touching and humorous memoir about the rewards and challenges he's experienced over the course of his running life. Yasso gives valuable advice on how to become a runner for life and continually draw joy from the sport. He also offers practical guidance for runners of all levels, including training schedules for 5-Ks, half-marathons, and marathons, all featuring his innovative speed-work technique known as Yasso 800s. His message: Never limit where running can take you, because each race has the potential for adventure.

Mile Markers
by Kristin Armstrong

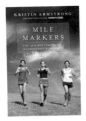

In *Mile Markers, Runner's World* contributing editor Kristin Armstrong captures the ineffable and timeless beauty of running, the importance of nurturing relationships with those we love, and the significance of reflecting on our experiences. With unique wit, refreshing candor, and disarming vulnerability, Armstrong shares her conviction that running is the perfect analogy for marking the milestones of life. Running threads together Armstrong's touching stories, and through each of them we are shown the universal undercurrents of inspiration, growth, grace, family, empowerment, and endurance. A perfect read for any woman who loves running.

The Long Run
by Matt Long with Charles Butler

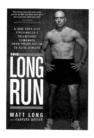

On the morning of December 22, 2005, New York City firefighter Matt Long was cycling to work when he was struck by and sucked under a 20-ton bus making an illegal turn. The injuries he sustained pushed him within inches of death. *The Long Run* is the emotional and honest story of Matt's determination to fight through fear, despair, and intense physical and psychological pain to regain the life he once had. It chronicles Matt's road to recovery as he teaches himself to walk again and, a mere 3 years later, to run the 2008 New York City Marathon. "Running saved my life," Matt says, and his embrace of the running community and insistence on competing in the marathon have inspired many, turning him into a symbol of hope and recovery.

The Athlete's Palate Cookbook: Renowned Chefs, Delicious Dishes, and the Art of Fueling Up While Eating Well
by Yishane Lee and the editors of *Runner's World* magazine

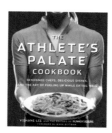

Training hard doesn't have to mean fueling up for workouts with flavorless foods. The all-star roster of chefs who contribute to the magazine's popular column "Athlete's Palate" include the likes of Bobby Flay, Jacques Torres, Charlie Trotter, Mark Bittman, Dan Barber, and Cat Cora.

With healthy and delicious recipes for all phases of training—along with quick-and-easy food tips, training, and recovery meals—this book is perfect for any athlete who wants to eat well.

The Runner's Field Manual: A Tactical (and Practical) Survival Guide
by Mark Remy and the editors of Runner's World

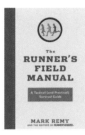

In this manual, more Boy Scout field guide than Emily Post's etiquette, you'll learn about everything from first aid (popping blisters) to navigation (sans GPS) to identifying species that runners may encounter on the road. Discover useful and entertaining advice on navigating water stops, crossing streets, and signing race waivers (you're better off not reading the fine print). Veteran runners will nod in recognition at the *Field Manual*'s lessons and asides, and newcomers will appreciate the insider info.

PHOTO CREDITS

NOTES

_____

_____

_____

_____

_____

_____

_____

_____

_____

_____

_____

_____

_____

_____